Insulin Therapy

Mark W.J. Strachan • Brian M. Frier

Insulin Therapy

A Pocket Guide

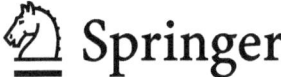 Springer

Mark W.J. Strachan, MD,
FRCP (Ed)
Metabolic Unit
Western General Hospital
Edinburgh
United Kingdom

Brian M. Frier, MD, FRCP,
(Ed and Glas)
BHF Centre for
Cardiovascular Science
The Queen's Medical Institute
University of Edinburgh
Edinburgh
United Kingdom

ISBN 978-1-4471-4759-6   ISBN 978-1-4471-4760-2   (eBook)
DOI 10.1007/978-1-4471-4760-2
Springer London Heidelberg New York Dordrecht

Library of Congress Control Number: 2013932841

Printed on acid-free paper

Springer is part of Springer Science+Business Media (www.springer.com)

Contents

Chapter 1
History, Normal Physiology, and Production of Insulin

Secretion, Physiology, and Metabolic Actions of Insulin in Humans

Insulin is produced in the pancreas, where it is secreted from beta cells located in the islets of Langerhans. The islets are surrounded by exocrine tissue but have a rich vascular and neural supply. Insulin-secreting beta cells constitute 85 % of the cells of the islets. The other endocrine cells—alpha and delta cells—produce the hormones glucagon and somatostatin, respectively, and pancreatic polypeptide is secreted from other cells. Insulin is synthesized and stored as proinsulin, which consists of two chains of amino acids, an A and B chain, joined by a connecting peptide, C-peptide (Fig. 1.1). C-peptide is split off by beta cell peptidases; insulin and C-peptide are secreted in equimolar amounts. Insulin is released into the portal circulation. An awareness of the relationship between insulin and C-peptide has practical applications, as manufactured insulin does not contain C-peptide. Measurement of C-peptide is, therefore, a useful way to differentiate between hypoglycemia secondary to exogenous insulin administration (plasma insulin is elevated; C-peptide is low or absent) and hypoglycemia secondary to endogenous hyperinsulinemia, as in the case of sulfonylurea excess or an insulinoma (insulin and C-peptide are both elevated).

The secretion of insulin is biphasic. In the first phase, insulin is released rapidly from stored vesicles in response to a rise of blood glucose following the consumption of food and

M.W.J. Strachan, B.M. Frier, *Insulin Therapy*,
DOI 10.1007/978-1-4471-4760-2_1,
© Springer-Verlag London 2013

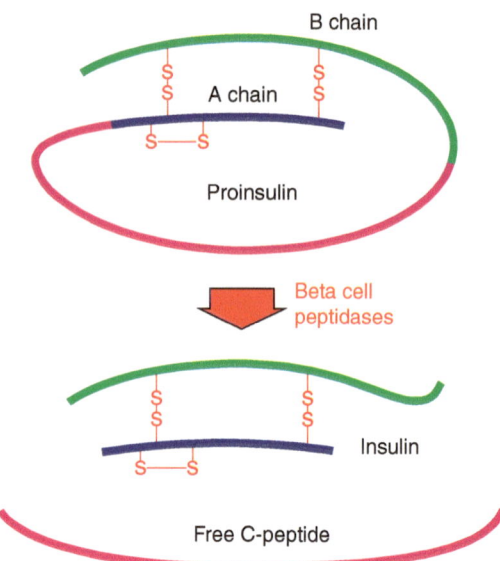

FIGURE 1.1 Structure of human proinsulin and insulin showing the alpha and beta chains and C-peptide

in response to other secretagogues, such as certain amino acids and hormones. In the second phase, new insulin is manufactured and released in a slow and sustained manner. Secretion of insulin is continuous and this background, or basal, secretion accounts for about 50 % of total daily production, occurring in regular pulses that are independent of blood glucose concentrations.

In humans insulin is the main anabolic hormone. The actions of insulin are summarized in Table 1.1; it promotes the uptake and storage of carbohydrate, amino acids, and fat into liver, skeletal muscle, and adipose tissue and antagonizes the catabolism of these fuel reserves. Insulin also has effects on cell growth, cognition, and the vasculature, which are separate from its metabolic actions. As insulin acts to increase glucose uptake and storage, blood glucose levels decline and secretion of insulin eventually stops. The half-life of insulin in the circulation is short—between 2 and 3 min. If glucose levels

TABLE 1.1 Actions of insulin

Increase (anabolic effects)	Decrease (anti-catabolic effects)
Carbohydrate metabolism	
Glycogenesis[a]	Glycogenolysis[a]
Glycolysis	Gluconeogenesis[a]
Glucose transport (muscle, adipose tissue, liver)	
Lipid metabolism	
Glycerol and triglyceride synthesis	Lipolysis
	Ketogenesis
Protein metabolism	
Protein synthesis	Protein degradation
Amino acid uptake	
Other actions	
Increase vascular compliance	
Enhance secretion of gastric acid	
Improve cognition (direct effect on neurons)	
Enhance cell growth and differentiation (mitogenic and antiapoptotic effects)	

[a]These actions reduce hepatic glucose output

fall below normal (hypoglycemia), several counterregulatory hormones are released. The most important are glucagon and adrenaline (epinephrine), which promote glycogenolysis and gluconeogenesis and so raise levels of glucose in the blood and restore normoglycemia. Other counterregulatory hormones include cortisol and growth hormone.

When insulin secretion is deficient or absent—as in people with type 1 diabetes—glucose accumulates in the blood and cannot be transported into peripheral tissues, which then seek an alternative source of energy. Uncontrolled gluconeogenesis and lipolysis lead to the development of metabolic decompensation and ketoacidosis.

Discovery, Isolation, and First Clinical Use of Insulin

In the 1870s, Bouchardat suggested an association between the pancreas and diabetes, which was confirmed a decade later when Minkowski and von Mering showed that diabetes developed in dogs when the pancreas was removed. In 1901, Opie established that the pancreatic islets of Langerhans were implicitly involved in the development of diabetes, and in 1910, Sharpey-Shafer suggested that the pancreas of diabetic patients was missing a single critical chemical, which, although then unidentified, he named "insulin."

Controversy surrounds the discovery of insulin, with many researchers such as Scott in the USA, Zuelzer in Germany, and the Romanian Paulesco, all coming close to discovering insulin. In 1921, the Canadians, Frederick Banting and his assistant Charles Best, working with a Scot, John Macleod, the Professor of Physiology at the University of Toronto, succeeded in lowering the high blood glucose of pancreatectomized dogs with diabetes by injecting them with pancreatic extracts from healthy dogs. In collaboration with the biochemist James Collip, they subsequently managed to prepare a relatively pure isolate which contained insulin from the pancreas of cattle.

In January 1922, the first successful administration of insulin was given to a patient with type 1 diabetes—Leonard Thomson—a 14-year-old youth in Toronto General Hospital. These pancreatic extracts were used subsequently to treat other diabetic patients with ketoacidotic coma in the hospital, and this heralded the onset of the insulin era for treating diabetes. Banting and Macleod were awarded the Nobel Prize for the discovery of insulin in 1923.

Milestones in Development of Insulin

Developments in the production of insulins have occurred at approximately 10-year intervals (Table 1.2) with various additives such as protamine and zinc, or the development of

TABLE 1.2 Milestones in the development of insulin

1920s	Isolation and development of soluble insulin
1930s	Long-acting insulins (protamine, zinc additives)
1940s	Isophane (NPH) insulins
1950s	Lente insulins
1970s	Purification of animal insulins
1980s	Human insulins
1990s	Insulin analogues
2000s	Biosimilar insulins

crystalline forms, slowing the absorption of insulin and providing longer-acting preparations. Human sequence insulin was introduced in the 1980s, and more recently analogues of human insulin have been developed, which have expanded the range and versatility of insulin regimens. Biosimilar insulins are now available.

Animal Insulins

Following the successful clinical use of insulin, efforts were intensified to improve the purity and upscale the production of bovine insulin. Initial attempts led to a higher yield, but the product remained impure. In early 1922, collaboration with the pharmaceutical company Eli Lilly led to large quantities of refined and relatively "pure" insulin becoming available for clinical use within 6 months. Insulin derived from pig pancreata subsequently became available, and in the subsequent decades, the purity of preparations steadily improved with the removal of islet peptides and other pancreatic constituents.

Long-Acting Insulins

Initially, insulin was available only in native form (so-called soluble or regular) and so had to be administered on multiple occasions each day. The next major development was in the production of delayed-action formulations. Initially these were tried without giving concurrent soluble insulin, until diabetologists better understood how they should be used effectively in clinical practice. The first of these was protamine insulate which was introduced by Hans Christian Hagedorn in Denmark in 1936. Subsequently, protamine zinc insulin, globin insulin, neutral protamine Hagedorn (NPH), and lente insulins became available.

Human Insulin

The full characterization of the amino acid sequence of human insulin by Sanger in 1955 and the subsequent discovery of the three-dimensional structure of the molecule by Hodgkin in 1969 led to the production of the first synthetic insulin from amino acids in the 1960s. In the late 1970s, genetically engineered synthetic human insulin was produced using recombinant DNA technology, and the first preparation became commercially available in 1982. Human insulin today is made using the recombinant DNA techniques first developed in the late 1970s. The first genetically engineered synthetic human insulin was made by inserting the gene that encodes for human insulin into the bacterium *Escherichia coli*. The process is similar today, in that the human gene is cloned and inserted into bacteria. Huge containers of the genetically modified bacteria can produce large quantities of human insulin, which is purified to provide pharmaceutical-grade pure human insulin or its analogues (Fig. 1.2).

Insulin Analogues

Advances in genetic engineering allowed manufacturers to alter the amino acid sequence of the insulin molecule to alter its pharmacokinetic properties and so create analogues of insulin; the first insulin "analogue," insulin lispro, which has a

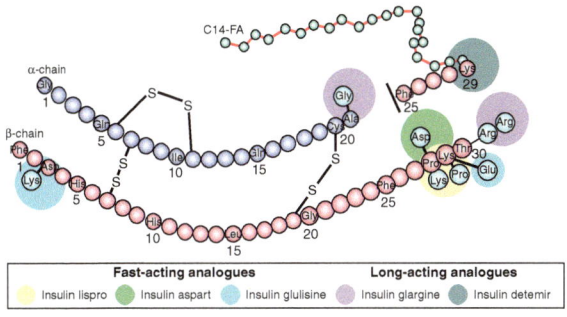

FIGURE 1.2 Analogues of human insulin

more rapid action than conventional soluble insulin, became available in the 1990s. Insulin analogues have also been developed which have a much slower rate of absorption and therefore a prolonged duration of action.

Stored insulin forms a biologically inactive hexameric structure, and when injected subcutaneously, the rate of onset of its action depends on how quickly it dissociates into active monomers. Human insulin has a faster onset of action than either of the animal-derived insulins (porcine insulin has a faster onset of action than bovine insulin). However, the older conventional soluble insulins have a relatively slow onset of action so that a patient should take these insulins about 30 min before eating food. The rapid-acting human insulin analogues, insulin lispro, insulin aspart, and insulin glulisine, have weak bonds between the monomeric components, enabling rapid dissociation of hexamers to monomers. These can then be absorbed rapidly from a subcutaneous injection site, and their hypoglycemic effect commences within 5–10 min. Conversely, long-acting insulin analogues—insulin glargine and insulin detemir—slowly dissociate and are slowly absorbed with only a modest peak of plasma insulin and have a protracted effect for 16–24 h. The plasma insulin concentrations associated with these long-acting analogues reach a plateau level, which persists for most of the day and more closely mimics basal secretion of insulin in the nondiabetic state. They are usually administered once or twice daily. Even longer-acting analogues, such as insulin degludec, last for up to 42 hours with no peak in activity.

Biosimilar Insulins

Biosimilars are generic versions of recombinant DNA technology drugs which are synthesized by a different manufacturing process. Unlike standard generic pharmaceuticals, drugs with a protein structure, like insulin, which are made by a different manufacturing process to the original drug may not be absolutely identical because there could be alterations in, for example, the quaternary (or folding) structure. Biosimilars cannot therefore be approved for clinical use by following the standard procedure as used for generic drugs, which requires simply the demonstration of equivalent bioavailability with the reference drug. Instead they have to pass strict mandates from pharmaceutical regulatory authorities. Biosimilars for human insulins have been developed and are in use in some parts of the world. Enthusiasm to prescribe such drugs has to be tempered by potential concerns about safety, quality, and comparable efficacy.

Chapter 2
Insulins and Regimens in Current Use

Indications for Insulin Therapy

Insulin is required to treat the following groups:

1. Type 1 diabetes (ketosis-prone) — all patients from diagnosis
2. Type 2 diabetes

   - With secondary failure to anti-diabetic drugs or poor glycemic control
   - During severe intercurrent illness (may be temporary)
   - With acute metabolic complications (e.g., hyperosmolar states)
   - With advanced diabetic complications, for example, renal failure
   - Before, during, and after surgery or major procedures
   - During treatment with oral or parenteral steroids (glucocorticoids)

3. Gestational diabetes (after failure with diet and or oral anti-diabetic drugs)

Types of Insulin

Insulins are classified by their duration of action into three main groups:

- Short-acting
- Intermediate-acting
- Long-acting

M.W.J. Strachan, B.M. Frier, *Insulin Therapy,*
DOI 10.1007/978-1-4471-4760-2_2,
© Springer-Verlag London 2013

Short-acting, unmodified insulin is called "soluble" insulin in the UK and "regular" insulin in North America and appears as a clear solution. The duration of action can be extended by the addition at neutral pH of a fish protein called protamine to form *isophane* (or *NPH* (neutral protamine Hagedorn)) insulin. Protamine binds with insulin and reduces its solubility after injection, so delaying its absorption. By adding an excess of zinc ions to insulin, crystallization of insulin in a suspension is produced, which will also delay release of insulin following subcutaneous injection. This forms *lente* insulins, which are suspensions of insulin zinc crystals. These modified "depot" insulins are cloudy preparations. Lente insulins have largely been superseded by modern insulins with more predictable time-action profiles, and their use has diminished in recent years. Very long-acting insulin (*Ultralente*) is now seldom used.

Most formulations of insulin in current use are identical to human insulin, being prepared biosynthetically from bacteria using recombinant DNA technology, but some patients prefer to use animal insulins (porcine and bovine), produced by extraction from animal pancreata. These insulins are described in Chap. 1 and examples are *Hypurin Bovine Neutral* (short-acting) and *Hypurin Porcine Isophane* (intermediate-acting), or insulin zinc suspension (e.g., *Hypurin Bovine Lente*), which is a neutral crystalline suspension of bovine and /or porcine insulin in a complex with zinc. These animal insulins have different time-action profiles from human insulins, with slower absorption characteristics and more prolonged hypoglycemic activity, and, because of differing amino acid sequences compared to human insulin, are more immunogenic and promote the formation of insulin antibodies. These features may be of value to some patients, such as those with impaired awareness of hypoglycemia or with gastroparesis, in whom a rapid fall in blood glucose can promote sudden and severe hypoglycemia. This is often a matter of personal choice, but it is important that access to animal insulins is maintained.

Insulin Analogues

By altering the amino acid sequence of insulin, it has been possible to produce insulin analogues, which differ in their rates of absorption from the site of injection. These comprise rapid-acting insulins and both intermediate-acting and long-acting insulins. Insulin analogues shown as the generic name with the trade name given in brackets that are currently available in the UK are:

- *Rapid-acting*:
  Insulin lispro (*Humalog*)
  Insulin aspart (*Novorapid*)
  Insulin glulisine (*Apidra*)
- *Intermediate-long-acting*:
  Insulin detemir (*Levemir*)
- *Long-acting*:
  Insulin glargine (*Lantus*)
  Insulin degludec (*Tresiba*)

It should be noted that unlike the conventional isophane or lente insulins, which are cloudy in appearance, the longer-acting analogues are all clear and cannot be distinguished visually from short- or rapid-acting insulins. The label on the vial or cartridge of insulin must always be checked before administration.

The time characteristics of insulins are shown in Table 2.1.

TABLE 2.1 Duration of action (in hours) of insulin preparations

Type of insulin	Onset	Peak	Duration
Rapid-acting			
lispro, aspart, glulisine	<0.25	0.5–2.5	3–6
Short-acting			
soluble (regular)	0.5–1	1–4	4–8
Intermediate-acting			
isophane (NPH), lente	1–3	3–8	7–14
detemir	1–3	3–12	7–18
Long-acting			
bovine ultralente	2–4	6–12	12–30
glargine	1–2	Minimal	18–24
degludec	1–2	None	42

The duration of action of any type of insulin varies considerably between individual patients, and some insulins (especially isophane) shows considerable intraindividual variability. This biological variation may account for some of the inconsistency of action of insulin in different patients.

Fixed Mixtures of Insulins

Premixed, or *biphasic*, formulations contain short-acting and intermediate-long-acting insulins in various proportions. Premixed insulins contain protamine insulin (intermediate-acting) and free insulin (short-acting). In Europe, the short-acting component is stated first (e.g., 30/70 contains 30 % of the short-acting component and 70 % of the intermediate-long-acting component) whereas in the USA, the opposite nomenclature is used (e.g., 70/30). The most commonly used mixture contains a combination of 30 % of a short-acting and 70 % of an intermediate-acting insulin (e.g., *Humulin M3*). Other combinations (e.g., 10:90 or 20:80) had limited usage and have been withdrawn by the manufacturers. Combinations of rapid-acting and intermediate- or long-acting insulin analogues in different proportions (e.g., *Humalog Mix 25*, *Humalog Mix 50*, or *Novomix 30*) are popular. All of these fixed mixtures have to be resuspended before injection by adequate agitation of the vial or cartridge containing the two insulins to ensure that the correct mixture is administered by the patient. Selection of an appropriate mixture has to be determined by the needs of the individual patient. Fixed mixtures have therapeutic limitations, particularly related to inability to adjust the doses of the individual components, and do not provide flexibility to accommodate daily changes in lifestyle or events.

In almost all countries, the insulin concentration in available formulations has been standardized at 100 units/ml (U-100). A high-strength insulin (*Humulin R U-500*) which contains 500 units/ml. can be obtained on a named basis for patients with severe insulin resistance, who require very large doses.

Subcutaneous Insulin Regimens

The choice of an insulin regimen is determined by various factors:

- Targets for glycemic control
- Time-action profile of the insulins to be used
- Ease and convenience of administration
- Flexibility in relation to lifestyle
- Practical issues (e.g., physical disability, ease of supply, species preference)

The insulin regimens that are in common use are:

1. *Basal-bolus* (*multiple injections*): Short-acting (or fast-acting) insulin is injected before meals (bolus), and an intermediate-acting or long-acting insulin is given once daily (basal). This regimen is suitable for both type 1 and type 2 diabetes.
    Examples are soluble insulin (e.g., *Actrapid* or *Humulin S*) before meals with isophane insulin (e.g., *Insulatard* or *Humulin I*) at bedtime or insulin aspart (*Novorapid*), insulin lispro (*Humalog*), or insulin glulisine (*Apidra*) before meals, with either insulin glargine (*Lantus*) or insulin detemir (*Levemir*) once or twice daily.
2. *Twice daily* (*biphasic*): Soluble or fast-acting and isophane (NPH) insulins are given in combination, either after free mixing or as a fixed mixture. This regimen can be used in both type 1 and type 2 diabetes.
    Examples are soluble insulin (e.g., *Actrapid* or *Humulin S*) and an isophane insulin (*Insulatard* or *Humulin I*) free mixed and given together twice daily—with breakfast and with the evening meal. Alternatively, a fixed mixture such as *Humulin M3*, *Humalog Mix 25*, or *Novomix 30* can be administered twice daily at the same meal times.
3. *Once daily* (*basal*): An intermediate-acting or long-acting insulin is given once daily (usually at bedtime) in combination with anti-diabetic drugs (used almost exclusively in patients with type 2 diabetes). Either an isophane insulin (e.g., *Insulatard* or *Humulin I*) or a long-acting insulin analogue (e.g., *Lantus* or *Levemir*) can be used. The main role

of insulin in this situation is to suppress hepatic release of glucose overnight and lower fasting blood glucose. This can be given with any of the oral anti-diabetic drugs. Many patients who require the addition of basal insulin are already taking multiple medications to which they may be developing secondary failure as their pancreatic beta cell function is progressively failing.

These insulin regimens are illustrated in Fig. 2.1, showing the time-action profiles of the individual insulins throughout 24 h. The basal-bolus regimen most closely simulates the physiological pattern of secretion of endogenous insulin in relation to the ingestion of food as it occurs in the nondiabetic state. It is very flexible as the timing of administration of the short- (or rapid-) acting insulin can be directly related to meals with additional doses being given with snacks if necessary. When a rapid-acting insulin analogue is used, it can be given before, during, or after food, in contrast to conventional soluble insulin, which has to be injected around 30 min before food to allow adequate time for absorption and onset of its hypoglycemic action.

With insulin analogues, the size and nature of the meal may be of importance with respect to the timing of insulin administration. In people with type 1 diabetes who have good glycemic control, the ingestion of a large meal (particularly when high in fat) slows gastric emptying, and if they have near-normoglycemia preprandially, it may be safer to administer a rapid-acting insulin analogue *after* the meal, to avoid provoking early hypoglycemia. Similarly, postprandial administration of a rapid-acting insulin analogue may be sensible if a meal contains a large proportion of carbohydrate in a slow-release (starch) form. Gastric emptying is delayed in many people with type 1 diabetes of long duration and is particularly severe in those with gastroparesis secondary to autonomic dysfunction, in whom rapid-acting insulin analogues should be avoided.

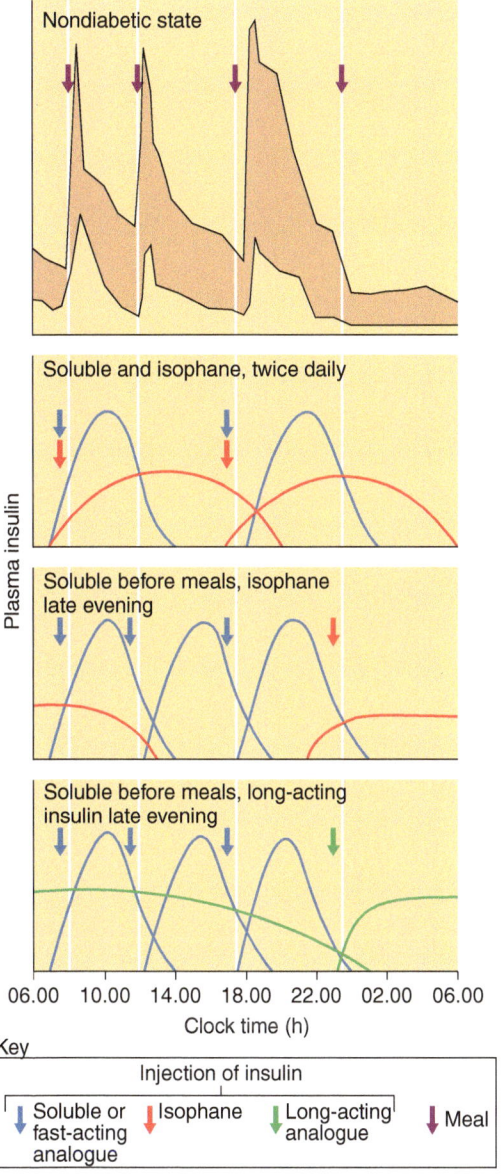

FIGURE 2.1 Insulin regimens

Chapter 3
Subcutaneous Insulin Administration

Insulin is administered mostly via the subcutaneous route. Because insulin is a protein, it is degraded by gastric secretions, and at present no oral formulations of insulin are commercially available. Insulin can be administered intravenously or by intramuscular injection, but these routes are reserved for treating metabolic emergencies or for specific management of hospital inpatients (Chaps. 6 and 7). Inhaled insulins were developed as a way of bypassing the gut. However, the only inhaled insulin to gain regulatory approval was withdrawn in 2007, because of fears about serious side effects. Insulin can be added to peritoneal dialysate, and implantable pumps in the abdominal wall can deliver insulin directly into the peritoneal cavity but are seldom used.

Many devices are available to deliver insulin subcutaneously. Some are specific to particular forms of insulin and have unique advantages and disadvantages. Ultimately, selection depends upon the type of insulin to be administered, individual preference, and cost.

Insulin Syringes

Since its discovery, insulin has been administered by subcutaneous injection using some form of syringe device and needle. Reusable metal syringes and needles were used for over 50 years but are cumbersome and require repeated sterilization, and injections are painful. They were replaced by a single-use plastic

M.W.J. Strachan, B.M. Frier, *Insulin Therapy*,
DOI 10.1007/978-1-4471-4760-2_3,
© Springer-Verlag London 2013

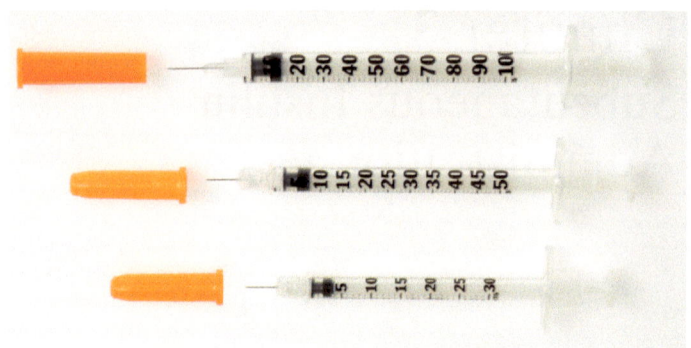

FIGURE 3.1 30 unit, 50 unit, and 100 unit insulin syringes

"insulin syringe" (Fig. 3.1), which is still widely used, particularly in low-resource economies and in hospitals. It has a fixed needle, is pre-sterilized, and can be used more than once if necessary. The syringes are available in different sizes—1 ml (100 units), 0.5 ml (50 units), and 0.3 ml (30 units)—with different needle lengths (12.7 and 8 mm) and diameters, 29 G (0.33 mm diameter), 30 G (0.30 mm diameter), and 31 G (0.26 mm).

Insulin Pens

The prototype of the insulin pen was developed in Scotland, and different versions emerged for clinical use in the 1980s. With increasing technological sophistication, pen devices have offered a simple and convenient means of administering subcutaneous insulin. A major advantage of the insulin pen is that the insulin is contained in a cartridge within the device, dispensing with the need to draw up insulin into a syringe from a vial. Disposable pens are discarded when the insulin cartridge is empty, while reusable pens deploy replaceable insulin cartridges (Figs. 3.2 and 3.3).

Needle attachments are screwed on to the pen device and are produced in different sizes—the smallest currently being 32 G diameter and 4 mm in length. The discomfort that can be

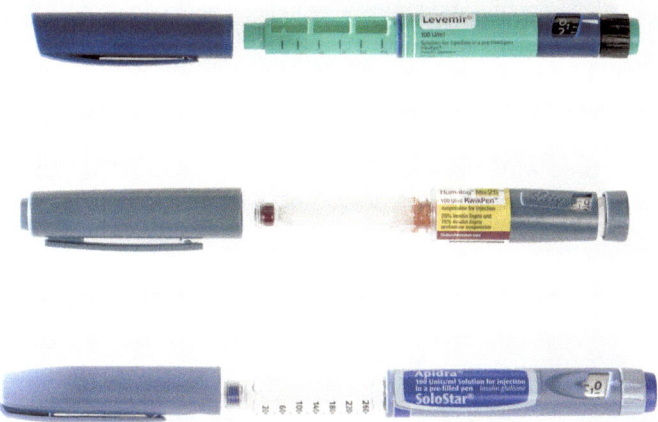

FIGURE 3.2 Disposable insulin pens

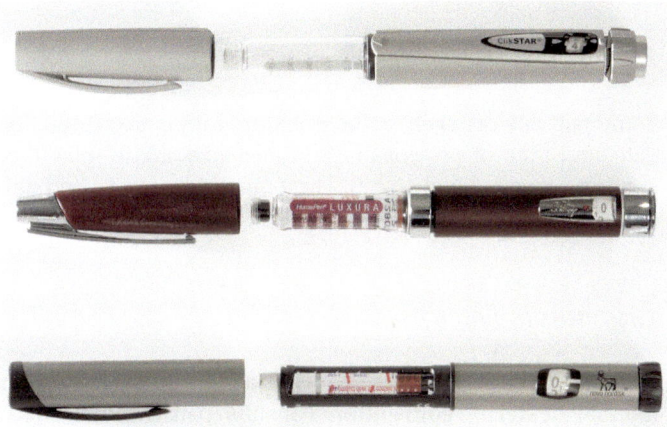

FIGURE 3.3 Reusable insulin pens

associated with insulin injection is reputed to be less than with a conventional syringe and needle, because the latter has not been partially blunted by prior insertion through the rubber diaphragm of an insulin vial and because pen needles are highly polished with a lubricant coating, for example, silicone.

Accuracy of dosing may be enhanced with pen devices by the capacity to dial the dose of insulin to be administered with precision. The insulin dose can be adjusted in increments of one unit, and some pens allow 0.5 unit adjustments. Most pens utilize a 3 ml cartridge (300 units of insulin) and the maximum deliverable dose with one injection ranges from 30 to 80 units. Safety refinements to most pen devices have made it impossible to dial and administer more insulin than remains in the cartridge.

All the commonly used insulins are available in pen devices. The choice of a particular brand of insulin within the same class may be influenced by the pen device available for that particular insulin. Aside from increased cost compared with reusable syringes, the main disadvantage of the insulin pen device is that it is not possible to free-mix insulins.

Variations on the Pen Devices

Digital Devices

Some pen devices, such as the *Memoir* (Lilly), record the dose, date, and time of previous insulin injections and display these data on a small digital screen. These provide a record and aide-mémoire of when and how much insulin has been administered.

Ergonomic Devices

For those who have problems with visual impairment and/or manual dexterity, conventional insulin pen devices may be difficult to use. To estimate the dose when drawing up insulin, people with visual impairment sometimes count the audible clicks of modified pens. Alternatively, the "InnoLet" (Novo Nordisk) device has a large "egg-timer" dial that is easier to read and to adjust the dose. It also has a plastic platform adjacent to the needle that provides stability for the device when it is pressed against the skin (Fig. 3.4). This device can be used only with *Insulatard* and *Levemir* insulins.

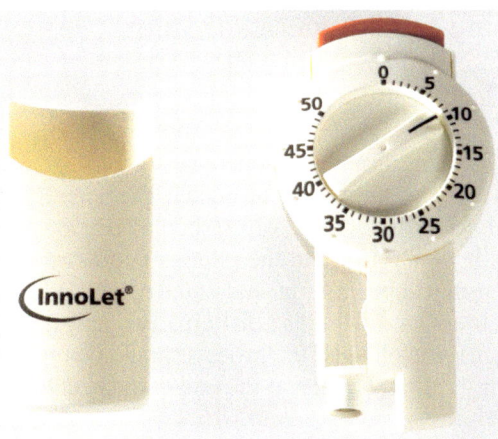

FIGURE 3.4 The Novo Nordisk InnoLet device has a large dial for people with visual impairment or manual dexterity problems. The plastic platform stabilizes the device when the needle is inserted into subcutaneous tissues

Needle-Free Devices

True needle phobia is rare, but for people who are unable to inject with a needle, needle-free devices are available that work by creating a fine jet of insulin that pierces the skin. They are often marketed as being "pain-free," but some discomfort at the injection site is common. They are also very noisy and their use is therefore much less discreet than conventional pens.

Storage of Insulin

Insulin vials, cartridges, and disposable pens should be refrigerated at 4 °C until required for use. Ideally, the insulin should be allowed to warm to room temperature before it is injected. Once a pen or cartridge is in use, it may be kept at room temperature for up to 30 days, following which any residual insulin should be discarded.

Injecting Subcutaneous Insulin

"Air Shots"

Before injecting insulin, patients are advised to make an "air shot" to expel air trapped in the needle. The potential to draw up air is greater with a syringe, which should be held vertically with the needle uppermost and the plunger depressed until a small bleb of insulin appears at the end of the needle. With insulin pen devices, users are advised to dial up a two unit dose of insulin and depress the plunger; the process should be repeated until a bleb of insulin can be seen at the end of the needle.

Injection Sites

Insulin can be injected into different anatomical sites – the anterior abdominal wall, the outer thighs, the buttocks, and the upper arms. The absorption rate of insulin differs at each site, being absorbed most quickly from the abdominal wall and least quickly from the lower limbs, although it could be increased from this site by exercise. Injection sites should be rotated to avoid the development of lipohypertrophy (see Chap. 5). In practice, the abdominal wall is the most convenient site because the injection may be administered relatively unobtrusively and has a large surface area in most individuals. When using a basal-bolus regimen, it may be prudent to keep injections site-specific for time of injection to avoid frequent changes in absorption kinetics causing variability in blood glucose excursions.

Resuspension of Cloudy Insulins

Insulins that are in suspension (cloudy insulins), that is, iso-phane and premixed insulins (including those containing rapid-acting insulin analogues), must be resuspended before injection. This is vital to ensure that the correct formulation is injected and to ensure stability of the absorption kinetics. Regrettably, this is often ignored or inadequately addressed.

Failure to resuspend isophane insulins can cause significant variability of action and particularly affects nocturnal plasma insulin concentrations. The insulin cartridge or vial should not be shaken vigorously, but should be repeatedly inverted until the suspension is uniformly cloudy. Soluble and all analogue insulins (including rapid- and long-acting types) are not in suspension so are clear in appearance and may be administered without agitation of the pen or vial.

Needle Length

Most people, even when obese, use 5 or 6 mm needles, and shorter (4 mm) needles are now available. With shorter needles, it is not necessary to pinch up the skin before injecting. The use of 12 and 12.7 mm needles is no longer necessary and risks intramuscular injection, which will alter insulin absorption. Pen needles and syringes should be changed following each injection and disposed of safely.

Injection Technique

Insulin should be injected at 90° to the surface of the skin. Patients are often advised to keep the needle in place for at least 10 s, to reduce leakage from the injection site when the needle is withdrawn. Bruising and discomfort at the site of an injection is usually a consequence of intramuscular injection. Pain at the injection site is unusual and may be caused by poor technique or failure to change the needle after each injection. Some preparations, particularly insulin glargine, are associated with a burning sensation following injection—this is related to the acid pH of the insulin solution.

Insulin Pumps

Delivery of insulin via a pump device, known as continuous subcutaneous insulin infusion (CSII), was developed in the 1960s and was first used with moderate but limited clinical

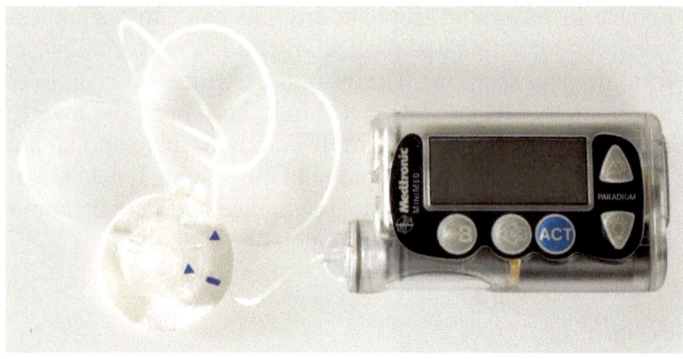

FIGURE 3.5 A Medtronic insulin pump with giving set and cannula

success in the subsequent two decades. Technological developments and safety refinements have encouraged more widespread use of insulin pumps, principally for the treatment of type 1 diabetes. An insulin pump is essentially a battery-operated syringe driver which administers insulin via a giving set which ends in a fine gauge plastic cannula which is sited subcutaneously, usually in the anterior abdominal wall (Fig. 3.5). A rapid-acting insulin analogue is the usual insulin of choice. A continuous "basal" amount of insulin is infused and a "bolus" dose may be administered at mealtimes.

The more sophisticated pumps are able to calculate how much "active insulin" will be in the recipient's body, and using algorithms can calculate an appropriate dose for the bolus, taking into account the patient's blood glucose, the amount of carbohydrate to be consumed in the next meal, and the patient's known insulin sensitivity. It is also possible to change the shape of the bolus wave, to accommodate the macronutrient content of a meal. Because a high-fat meal delays gastric emptying, an "extended square wave" may be employed; some patients use a "dual wave" (which has two peaks) for a meal with a high starch content.

Correction of postprandial or pre-bedtime hyperglycemia with additional bolus injections of rapid-acting insulin is discouraged because of the difficulty of estimating the dose of insulin with accuracy, and this practice risks hypoglycemia. However, the ability of the pump to calculate the amount of "active" insulin has made the decision on appropriate insulin doses for correction boluses more scientific and safer. It is possible to give correction doses as low as 0.025 units.

While the absolute dose of basal insulin using conventional regimens may be adjusted upward or downward, it is not possible to vary the time-action profile. By contrast, the rate of infusion of basal insulin at any time point can be varied using a pump. It is possible to program the pump to administer a higher dose of basal insulin at predetermined times, for example, between 04.00 and 08.00 h to counteract the "dawn phenomenon" of fasting hyperglycemia. By contrast, if an individual is prone to hypoglycemia during the night, the overnight basal insulin rate can be reduced. For periods of physical activity, such as vigorous exercise, pumps have the facility to introduce a lower "temporary basal rate." A higher "temporary basal rate" can be used during periods of intercurrent illness. The marked day-to-day variability that is common with isophane insulins does not occur with CSII, presumably because the insulin is given continuously at low doses and is not being absorbed from a subcutaneous depot.

In an appropriately motivated patient, these factors can provide a more physiological pattern of insulin delivery than can be obtained with conventional subcutaneous injections and diminishes blood glucose excursions. Glycemic control can be improved without increasing the risk of severe hypoglycemia. "Closed-loop" systems that integrate the insulin pump with data from a continuous subcutaneous monitor are under development. The key to their success will be in the development of algorithms that allow pump settings and insulin infusion rates to be altered in response to the glucose data.

Indications for Insulin Pump Therapy

CSII is considerably more expensive than conventional insulin administration and has received intense scientific and health economic scrutiny. The UK National Institute for

TABLE 3.1 NICE indications for CSII

CSII is recommended as a treatment option in type 1 diabetes

(a) For adults and children 12 years of age and over when either attempts to achieve target HbA1c levels with multiple daily insulin injections (MDI) result in disabling hypoglycemia or HbA1c levels remain high (≥8.5 % or 69 mmol/mol) on MDI therapy (including, if appropriate, the use of long-acting analogues of insulin) despite a high level of care

(b) For children younger than 12 years when MDI is considered to be impractical or inappropriate and with the expectation that children would be expected to undergo a later trial of MDI between the ages of 12 and 18 years

Health and Clinical Excellence (NICE) has published guidance on the indications for CSII in type 1 diabetes (Table 3.1). Initiation and ongoing support for people using insulin pumps requires considerable expertise and time from diabetes healthcare professionals, and CSII should be initiated by a trained specialist team. It is not currently recommended for people with type 2 diabetes.

Disadvantages and Risks of Insulin Pump Therapy

Acceptability

The insulin pump can be removed when bathing/showering or when swimming but otherwise has to be in continuous use. Many with type 1 diabetes do not wish to be attached to a pump for every hour of their lives, and this may be a difficult issue for young people. An insulin pump demands much greater effort on the part of the user, requiring carbohydrate counting at mealtimes, regular blood glucose testing, and frequent adjustment of the pump settings. Appropriate patient selection for CSII is essential.

Diabetic Ketoacidosis

The main danger of insulin pump therapy is DKA. This can develop rapidly if the insulin pump becomes disconnected or malfunctions or the tubing is occluded because no depot of basal insulin is available to prevent ketosis. An alarm will sound if the giving set is occluded or if insulin in the reservoir becomes low, but the alarm will not be activated if the pump is disconnected, for example, if the cannula is dislodged or incorrectly sited, because the pump cannot detect any abnormal increase in infusion pressure. Users are given very strict instructions to monitor their blood glucose carefully, particularly after changing a giving set, and to check blood or urine ketone concentrations if hyperglycemia ensues. "Sick-day" rules must also be closely adhered to, with insulin infusion rates being increased during intercurrent illness. Users of CSII are advised to keep pens or vials of subcutaneous insulin available for injection in case of a pump malfunction.

Infections

Localized infections can occur at the site of the cannula, which should be changed at least every 3 days.

Management of insulin pumps in hospital inpatients is discussed in Chap. 7.

Chapter 4
Initiating and Adjusting Insulin

Treatment with insulin is not a precise science!!! Many different types of insulins and insulin regimens are employed (Chap. 2). The choice of an insulin regimen will ultimately depend on an individual's lifestyle, ability to administer and cope with insulin therapy, and their likely compliance. In this chapter the practical steps to be taken in initiating insulin therapy and how to adjust insulin doses in people on insulin therapy are considered.

Initiation of Insulin Therapy

The process of commencing insulin therapy requires knowledge, expertise, and empathy. For the patient with newly diagnosed type 1 diabetes, there may be considerable emotional upset at the diagnosis of diabetes and its long-term implications, and treatment is usually commenced against a background of general malaise and metabolic derangement associated with this diagnosis. In some instances, insulin therapy will be started while the individual is recovering in hospital from diabetic ketoacidosis; in individuals with limited metabolic disturbance, insulin therapy may be initiated as an outpatient. This can be a turbulent and confusing time for the patient, and their family and the education process will generally be performed over several days, with a combination of face-to-face sessions and telephone contact. Written instructions are also necessary, as it is very difficult for

M.W.J. Strachan, B.M. Frier, *Insulin Therapy,*
DOI 10.1007/978-1-4471-4760-2_4,
© Springer-Verlag London 2013

patients to absorb and remember this torrent of new information. In people with type 2 diabetes, insulin is seldom commenced with such urgency, thus allowing the recipient time to adjust psychologically to the imminent need for insulin. Nevertheless, it may still be a time of emotional stress for the individual.

While the requirement for insulin is absolute in type 1 diabetes, the decision to commence insulin in a person with type 2 diabetes is not always so clear-cut. Many with type 2 diabetes will not be commenced on insulin therapy until several years after diagnosis, although by that time some patients may have experience of using other injectable preparations (GLP-1 analogues). The potential benefits have to be balanced against the principal risks of hypoglycemia and weight gain (Chap. 5). In an individual with very poorly controlled diabetes, insulin therapy will relieve osmotic symptoms and may permit the cessation of some tablets. Although good glycemic control will reduce the risk of developing vascular complications of diabetes, this may be less important in an older individual where symptom control and avoidance of hypoglycemia take precedence. General frailty and disability such as poor vision may prevent self-administration of insulin, and others such as district nurses or care home workers may be required to inject insulin. A decision has to be made regarding the most appropriate insulin regimen for the individual and in people with type 2 diabetes, which (if any) oral anti-diabetic agents should be discontinued.

Information to Be Imparted in the Insulin Initiation Education Sessions

The education sessions at the time of insulin initiation must address several issues:

- To provide information on the causes, treatment, and possible long-term effects of diabetes to newly diagnosed patients and to update patients with established diabetes

- To ensure that the patient can administer insulin safely
- To inform patients how to adjust the doses of insulin in relation to blood glucose measurements, food, and lifestyle, especially exercise and drinking alcohol
- To teach patients how to perform home blood glucose monitoring and how to recognize and treat hypoglycemia
- To teach patients with type 1 diabetes how to test for ketones, in urine or blood, and how to interpret and act on these results
- To provide advice on how to manage intercurrent illness and elevated blood glucose

A recommended checklist of specific topics to be covered is shown in Table 4.1. It may not be necessary to address all of these issues with every individual, particularly older people with type 2 diabetes and those who will not be self-administering insulin, but the quantity of information to be conveyed in a short time is potentially vast and may be intimidating. Typically, such education sessions will be performed by diabetes specialist nurses, with contributions from dietitians and podiatrists.

Factors Affecting Insulin Requirements

The dose of insulin required on a daily basis varies greatly between individuals and is mainly a consequence of differential insulin sensitivity. People with greater central obesity are usually more insulin resistant and require more insulin than lean individuals. Even on an individual basis, significant day-to-day variations can occur in insulin requirement. The consumption of carbohydrate and the intake of other foods also have a major influence on the amount of insulin required and will be modified by other factors such as exercise, alcohol intake, and intercurrent illness. Insulin-specific factors (Chap. 3) such as the site and depth of injection and the resuspension of isophane insulins also affect blood glucose profiles. Larger doses of insulin may peak later and last for longer than smaller doses and factors that increase subcutaneous blood

TABLE 4.1 Checklist for initiating insulin

What is diabetes?	Dietetic advice, including carbohydrate counting, if appropriate
Practical skills	*Hypoglycemia*
Pen type/syringe size	Symptoms
Injection technique	Causes
Storage of insulin	Treatment
Disposal of needles	How to administer glucagon
Needle length	Identity tags/bracelet/necklace
Information about insulin	*Blood glucose monitoring*
Insulin type	Meter type and operation
Action/duration	Finger pricking
Timing and number of injections	Timing of tests/frequency
Hyperglycemia	Target levels
Symptoms	Documentation of results/ downloading of data
Importance of good glycemic control	*Adjusting insulin therapy*
Relation to HbA1c	Exercise
Causes	Alcohol
Ketostix/blood ketone monitoring (type 1 diabetes)	Stress
"Sick-day" rules	
Living with diabetes and complications	
Contraception/pregnancy	Erectile dysfunction
Work	Travel
Alcohol	Foot care
Recreational drug use	Clinic appointments
Driving	Register for free prescriptions
Informing DVLA and motor insurance company	Diabetes UK
Eye screening	Useful websites (for sport and exercise see www.runsweet.com)

flow (exercise, local massage, and elevated skin temperature (e.g., following hot baths or saunas) may also enhance
absorption).

Insulin Doses at Initiation

Given the intra- and interindividual variation in insulin
requirements, determining the initial starting dose of insulin
can be difficult and may involve a degree of clinical trial and
some educated guesswork!

Type 1 Diabetes

People with established type 1 diabetes typically require 0.5–
0.7 units of insulin/kg body weight/day, but in a newly diagnosed patient, this requirement is often much lower
(approximately 0.2–0.5 units/kg/day) because of residual
endogenous insulin production. For an individual with type 1
diabetes who has been admitted to hospital, some indication
of the daily insulin requirement may be derived from the
amount of intravenous insulin that has been required.
However, this must be tempered by the fact that oral caloric
intake may have been low and that high doses of insulin may
have been required to overcome hyperglycemia and severe
acidosis. A long-acting insulin can be given initially while the
patient is still receiving i.v. insulin, and a similar approach can
be taken with an individual who is commencing insulin as
an outpatient. In adults, around 6–10 units of long-acting insulin can be administered initially and the effects on blood glucose observed over the subsequent 24 h. Diabetologists vary
in their practice in this situation—some prescribe soluble or a
rapid-acting insulin analogue immediately, while others commence a twice daily fixed mixture of insulin or may persevere
for longer with long-acting insulin. The patient may go into
remission (a so-called honeymoon period) for several months
and has a very low insulin requirement until their endogenous
insulin secretion declines and eventually ceases, during which
the insulin requirement rises progressively.

Type 2 Diabetes

Most national guidelines recommend that people with type 2 diabetes who are converted from oral medication to insulin therapy are commenced initially on a once daily injection of isophane (NPH) or a long-acting insulin analogue, usually given at bedtime. There is no difference between the two types of insulin with respect to lowering HbA1c, but the (more expensive) long-acting analogues may incur a lower risk of nocturnal hypoglycemia. Unless the patient has prominent osmotic symptoms, high-dose therapy is rarely needed initially, and most algorithms suggest starting with a low dose of insulin and titrating upward according to fasting blood glucose values. An initial start-up dose of 10 units at bedtime (or 0.1–0.2 units/kg) is commonly employed, and the dose can be increased by 2–5 units every 3 days until the fasting blood glucose reaches target. Metformin and sulfonylurea therapies are often continued, while other agents may be withdrawn.

If glycemic control remains suboptimal, then the introduction of prandial insulin may be necessary. This will either be in the form of a twice daily fixed mixture or as a basal-bolus regimen. Fixed mixtures are traditionally administered with two-thirds of the total daily dose before breakfast and one-third before the evening meal. This is an approximate guide, and the choice of mixture and dosing should be determined by appropriate blood glucose targets and the patient's lifestyle. If in doubt, insulin should be started at a low dose and gradually increased.

Adjusting Insulin Doses

Home Blood Glucose Monitoring (HBGM)

Regular HBGM is essential for people with insulin-treated diabetes. It is only by determining the glucose levels that rational adjustment of the insulin dose is possible. HBGM is also crucial to detect and confirm hypoglycemia; this is particularly important in people with long-duration type 1 diabetes who have impaired awareness of hypoglycemia. Although less common, impaired awareness of hypoglycemia may also develop in individuals with insulin-treated type 2 diabetes. Furthermore, the elderly have more difficulty in recognizing hypoglycemia so the possibility of asymptomatic hypoglycemia should not be overlooked in this group. Many different blood glucose meters are available, and as with insulin pens, the device used will depend on patient preference and, in some instances, economic factors.

The frequency of monitoring depends on the circumstances of the individual. An elderly person with type 2 diabetes who has a very constant routine with respect to meal times, meal content, and daily physical activity is likely to have stable and consistent insulin requirements, and frequent blood glucose testing may be unnecessary. Similarly, in a frail individual in whom hypoglycemia must be avoided and strict glycemic control is contraindicated, frequent HBGM is not justified. By contrast, individuals with impaired hypoglycemia awareness and/or have a very variable lifestyle may need or wish to measure blood glucose frequently. Such individuals are often using an advanced insulin regimen (basal-bolus or CSII).

In recent years, several types of continuous glucose monitor have become available. These measure interstitial glucose, usually in the subcutaneous tissue of the anterior abdominal wall. Some can download the result directly to an insulin pump and have an alarm that can be set to alert patients when glucose levels are too low or too high. At present, these devices are not funded through the NHS, but they have potential to improve the quality of glycemic control.

Target Glucose Levels

Glucose targets need to be chosen depending upon the individual circumstances of the patient. To achieve strict glycemic control in an individual with type 1 diabetes, premeal targets of 5–7 mmol/l are necessary. The target for pre-bed blood glucose should be higher at around 6–8 mmol/l, to lessen the risk of nocturnal hypoglycemia. Postprandial monitoring is advocated for patients using CSII and in some patients on a basal-bolus regimen, and a target of <10 mmol/l is often advocated. Higher target levels are invariably recommended for elderly people to reduce the risk of hypoglycemia.

Advanced Insulin Therapy Dose Adjustment

In recent years a sea change has occurred in the advice given to people with type 1 diabetes who are using more advanced insulin regimens (basal-bolus and CSII). This has resulted from the increased usage and sophistication of insulin pumps and the success of structured education programs such as DAFNE (Dose Adjustment For Normal Eating). Traditionally, patients were advised to adjust insulin doses on the basis of their glucose profiles the previous day, taking into account the nature of the meal to be consumed. This is still the preferred method for simpler insulin regimens and to adjust subcutaneous insulin therapy for people in hospital and is discussed later. What insulin pump therapy and structured education programs have demonstrated is that glycemic control can be improved and risk of hypoglycemia lowered by adjusting insulin doses on the basis of a semiquantitative assessment of mealtime carbohydrate content, a patient's estimated insulin sensitivity, and their prevailing blood glucose levels.

Carbohydrate Counting

Individuals with type 1 diabetes, where appropriate, are taught to adjust their mealtime insulin doses according to the estimated amount of carbohydrate in that meal. On average, one carbohydrate portion (10 g) raises blood glucose by

2–3 mmol/l. Most patients require approximately 1 unit of insulin for every 10 g carbohydrate portion. This often varies between individuals, and some people may find that they require to alter the insulin:carbohydrate ratio depending on the time of day. Ratios may be determined by keeping a food diary and by monitoring postprandial blood glucose. If the ratio is appropriate, the postprandial glucose should be no more than 3 mmol/l above the premeal value. A rough approximation of the likely insulin:carbohydrate ratio may be derived by using the "rule of 500"—that is, divide 500 by the total daily insulin dose. The resulting figure should be rounded to the nearest 5. For example, a patient takes 65 units of insulin/day, and the insulin:carbohydrate ratio is 500/65 = 7.7. This figure is rounded to 10, that is, the patient should administer 1 unit of insulin per 10 g carbohydrate in a meal.

No premeal insulin is required if the patient misses a meal (providing the basal rate is appropriate), and with CSII and rapid-acting analogue insulins, there is no requirement for a between-meal snack.

Insulin Sensitivity

The amount of insulin taken at mealtimes should be adjusted according to the prevailing blood glucose level. Patients are taught to determine how much 1 unit of insulin will lower their blood glucose (insulin sensitivity factor), in the absence of food. Once more this may be determined by reference to HBGM data, but as a rough guide, the "rule of 100" may be used—that is, divide 100 by the total daily insulin dose. In the patient above, the sensitivity factor is 1.5, that is, 1 unit of insulin lowers blood glucose by approximately 1.5 mmol/l. Box 4.1 shows some worked examples of how insulin:carbohydrate ratio and sensitivity factor should be used to determine a mealtime insulin dose.

Box 4.1: Examples of Determining Mealtime Insulin Requirements in a Patient Using Advanced Insulin Therapy

Patient A:	Patient B:
Insulin:carbohydrate ratio = 1:15	Insulin:carbohydrate ratio = 1:10
Insulin sensitivity factor = 3	Insulin sensitivity factor = 2
Premeal glucose = 10 mmol/l	Premeal glucose = 12 mmol/l
Target glucose 7 mmol/l	Target glucose 6 mmol/l
Meal estimated carbohydrate = 60 g	Meal estimated carbohydrate = 110 g
60/15 = 4 unit insulin required to cover meal carbohydrate	110/10 = 11 unit insulin required to cover meal carbohydrate
(10–7)/3 = 1 unit insulin required to correct glucose to target	(12–6)/2 = 3 unit insulin required to correct glucose to target
Total mealtime dose = 5 units	Total mealtime dose = 14 units

Correction Doses

Conventionally, patients were taught to avoid taking "extra" doses of insulin between meals, because this insulin may accumulate and be superimposed on the previous mealtime dose and potentially encourage hypoglycemia. Some insulin pumps have the facility to track the amount of "active insulin" in a patient's system and can make a scientific recommendation on whether this is appropriate and to make a correction dose based also on the patient's sensitivity factor and target glucose levels. This may also help to improve overall glycemic control.

Basal Insulin Dose Adjustment

In most individuals, the basal insulin requirement is approximately 50 % of the total daily insulin dose. The basal insulin dose is determined by the fasting blood glucose level. CSII offers the facility to alter the basal insulin rates during a 24-h cycle according to blood glucose profiles. The accuracy of the daytime infusion rates can be assessed by asking patients to omit a meal, or take a carbohydrate free meal, and by assessing blood glucose 2 hourly until the next meal. Thus, for example, if a patient takes a high-protein breakfast and has above target glucose levels throughout the morning, this is an indication to increase the morning basal infusion rate.

Conventional Insulin Therapy Dose Adjustment

Patients are usually instructed to adjust insulin doses with reference to the blood glucose levels the previous day that correspond to the time-action profile of the insulin injection in question. Thus, for a patient using a basal-bolus regimen, the breakfast bolus should be adjusted on the basis of the pre-lunch glucose on the previous day; the lunch bolus on the basis of the preceding glucose before the evening meal; the evening meal bolus on the basis of the previous pre-bed glucose; and the bedtime basal insulin on the basis of the preceding pre-breakfast glucose. A similar principle holds for fixed mixture insulins, such that the breakfast dose is adjusted on the basis of the preceding pre-lunch and pre-evening meal glucose values (with the rapid-acting component primarily affecting pre-lunch glucose and the long-acting the pre-evening meal glucose). The evening meal dose is adjusted on the basis of the pre-bed and pre-breakfast glucose (with the rapid-acting component influencing the pre-bed glucose and the long-acting insulin affecting the pre-breakfast glucose). Isolated high or low blood glucose values should not necessarily provoke an alteration in insulin dose, particularly if there was an obvious reason for the abnormal glucose reading, such as a missed meal or insulin injection. Furthermore, hyperglycemia can sometimes be a triggered by treatment or overtreatment of hypoglycemia, so the cause of erratic readings should be sought where possible.

Dose adjustments are usually made in 2–4 unit increments or decrements, although if a patient is very insulin resistant and takes over 100 units/day, larger individual dose adjustments have to be made. Conversely, in a very insulin-sensitive patient, 1 unit adjustments may be more appropriate. Additional insulin may be administered if the blood glucose is high or if the meal to be consumed is high in carbohydrate. If the patient is hypoglycemic at the time an insulin injection is due, they are advised not to omit the injection, but to eat the meal and administer the insulin some time afterwards when the low blood glucose has been corrected.

Examples of subcutaneous insulin dose adjustment are shown in Chap. 7.

Exercise

Exercise can have pronounced effects on blood glucose and, in particular, may lower blood glucose several hours later, causing "delayed" hypoglycemia. Adjustment of the insulin dose depends on the nature, intensity, and duration of the exercise. Prolonged exercise, such as hill walking or long-distance running, requires a reduction in total insulin dose (basal and preprandial) to prevent hypoglycemia. Short-duration intensive exercise, such as racket sports or sprinting, may not require alterations in insulin dose, but additional fast-acting (refined) carbohydrate should be consumed. If the exercise is planned, it is usually preferable to reduce the amount of insulin beforehand. If the exercise is unpremeditated, it is usually necessary to consume some fast-acting carbohydrate. Blood glucose should be checked at intervals if exercise is prolonged and should be monitored carefully afterwards. By doing so, patients can ascertain how they respond to exercise and can make rational decisions on insulin dose adjustment and/or appropriate carbohydrate intake.

Patients with type 1 diabetes are usually advised to avoid exercise if blood glucose concentrations are >14 mmol/l. Apart from hyperglycemia impairing exercise performance, the relative insulin deficiency associated with such a high blood glucose could lead to an increased risk of ketoacidosis through impairment of exercise-associated glucose utilization and increased hepatic glucose output in response to counter-regulatory hormone release. In such circumstances, individuals should be advised to take a correction dose of insulin and to defer exercise until blood glucose has been reduced.

Alcohol

Alcohol inhibits hepatic gluconeogenesis and can provoke hypoglycemia; therefore, it is usually not necessary to count the carbohydrate content of alcohol when determining meal-time insulin doses. Some alcoholic beverages such as beers and lagers have a high carbohydrate content, and some people observe a rise in their blood glucose after imbibing, such that a small increment in preprandial insulin dose may be required. However, this should be effected with caution, particularly if alcohol intake is associated with increased physical activity. Drinking alcohol without food is more likely to lead to delayed hypoglycemia (often nocturnal), and it may be necessary to reduce insulin doses before consuming alcohol to reduce the risk of delayed hypoglycemia.

Chapter 5
Side-Effects of Insulin

The most common side-effect of insulin therapy is hypoglycemia (low blood glucose), which is potentially serious and can be life-threatening; other complications of insulin therapy include weight gain, injection site abnormalities, and, rarely, insulin allergy.

Hypoglycemia

Hypoglycemia is a major adverse side-effect of insulin treatment and is the principal barrier to achieving and maintaining optimal glycemic control. While intensive treatment with insulin and sulfonylureas can achieve strict glycemic control and limit the risk of vascular complications in both type 1 and type 2 diabetes, it also exposes patients to the risk of developing hypoglycemia.

Symptoms and Pathophysiological Changes in Hypoglycemia

Symptoms of hypoglycemia are generated by activation of the sympathoadrenal system (autonomic symptoms) and through the effects of glucose deprivation on the brain (neuroglycopenic symptoms). The commonest symptom in young adults have been identified and classified as:

M.W.J. Strachan, B.M. Frier, *Insulin Therapy,*
DOI 10.1007/978-1-4471-4760-2_5,
© Springer-Verlag London 2013

- *Autonomic* — sweating, palpitations, shaking, hunger
- *Neuroglycopenic* — confusion, lack of coordination, drowsiness, unusual behavior, difficulty with speech
- *Nonspecific malaise* — headache, nausea

These symptoms are triggered when blood glucose falls below a threshold level, which is reproducible in nondiabetic people but can vary in people with diabetes as it is influenced by factors such as exposure to preceding hypoglycemia or the quality of glycemic control. Symptomatic responses to hypoglycemia are idiosyncratic and vary considerably from person to person, as well as varying between events. An individual has to be able to identify the onset of hypoglycemia to allow early corrective action by taking oral glucose; experienced patients can also anticipate their susceptibility at certain times or in particular circumstances, for example, after missing a meal or following strenuous exercise. The pattern of symptoms varies with age; the most common symptoms in children are associated with behavioral changes, while older people experience neurological symptoms, including visual disturbance, incoordination, and ataxia. The symptoms are similar whether hypoglycemia is induced by insulin or a sulfonylurea and are modified by age, but not the type of diabetes.

Classification, Frequency, and Causes of Hypoglycemia

The most useful clinical categorization of hypoglycemia is based on a patient's ability to self-treat and is defined as "mild" if this is possible and "severe" if external help is necessary, whether or not coma occurs. Neither the intensity nor nature of the symptoms, nor the type of treatment used, is of importance in defining severity.

Mild hypoglycemia occurs in people with type 1 diabetes approximately twice weekly on average; severe hypoglycemia has an annual prevalence of around 30 % in people with type 1 diabetes, and the incidence ranges from one episode per year to over three per year in those with diabetes of long duration (>15 years). Severe hypoglycemia occurs less frequently in people with insulin-treated type 2 diabetes but increases the longer a patient is on insulin therapy. The annual prevalence is around 7 % in the first 2 years of insulin therapy (similar to that observed with SUs) but rises to 25 % when patients have been treated with insulin for more than 5 years.

Hypoglycemia can be caused by:

- Too much insulin
- Inadequate intake of food or delayed meals
- Exercise
- Alcohol

An episode of hypoglycemia often has multifactorial causes, and in many instances of severe hypoglycemia, no specific cause can be identified.

Risk Factors for Hypoglycemia

The major risk factors for hypoglycemia are impaired awareness of hypoglycemia (see below), a history of previous severe hypoglycemia, strict glycemic control, increasing age and duration of diabetes, sleep, renal impairment, and loss of endogenous insulin production (C-peptide negativity).

Impaired Awareness of Hypoglycemia

Impaired awareness of hypoglycemia (IAH) is an acquired syndrome associated with recurrent exposure to hypoglycemia, in which affected individuals have progressive difficulty in perceiving the onset of the warning symptoms of hypoglycemia. These diminish in intensity over time and change in nature so that autonomic symptoms are lost and neuroglycopenic symptoms then predominate. As a consequence of adaptation of the brain to function at lower blood glucose levels than normal, symptoms are not triggered until blood glucose is very low. This does not allow adequate time for the individual to take corrective action to reverse the low blood glucose; cognitive function is impaired, neuroglycopenia supervenes, and rapid progression to severe hypoglycemia can then occur. The prevalence of IAH is around 20–25 % in type 1 diabetes and increases with duration of the disorder; almost 50 % of patients have developed IAH, and after 25 years the prevalence is less common in patients with insulin-treated type 2 diabetes (<10 %). The frequency of severe hypoglycemia is three to six times greater than in people with normal awareness.

Strategies that may be adopted to reduce the risk of severe hypoglycemia include:

- Frequent blood glucose monitoring.
- Avoid blood glucose falling below 4.0 mmol/l.
- Revise target glycemic levels upward and avoid HbA1c being maintained close to the nondiabetic range.
- Use short-acting insulins or insulin analogues in a basal-bolus regimen.
- Take frequent snacks containing unrefined carbohydrate.
- Continuous subcutaneous insulin infusion (insulin pump).

Management and Prevention of Hypoglycemia

The major challenge in the long-term management plan for people with diabetes is to minimize hypoglycemia while maintaining satisfactory glycemic control to limit complications. Early identification of a fall in blood glucose is fundamental in protecting against the risk of hypoglycemia, and regular blood glucose monitoring is essential. However, asymptomatic biochemical hypoglycemia is common, and its detection depends on frequent testing. Another key element in prevention is patient education. The recommended "four is the floor" by Diabetes UK reminds people treated with insulin that the lowest acceptable level of blood glucose should be 4.0 mmol/l.

Treatment of hypoglycemia is dependent upon the severity of the episode and ranges from oral ingestion of a carbohydrate snack or glucose drink to intensive parenteral treatment.

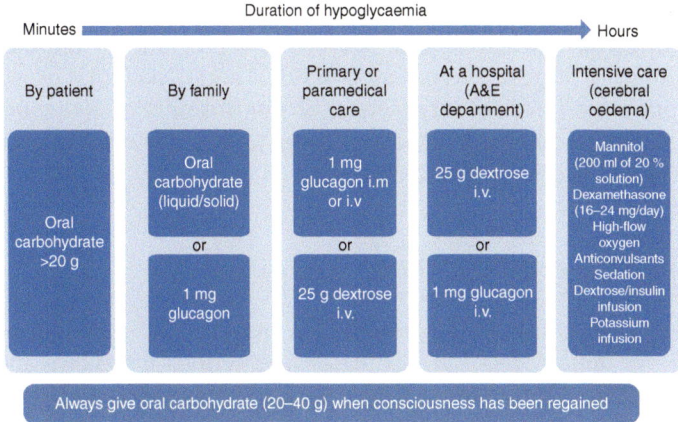

Duration of hypoglycaemia

Minutes ➡ Hours

By patient	By family	Primary or paramedical care	At a hospital (A&E department)	Intensive care (cerebral oedema)
Oral carbohydrate >20 g	Oral carbohydrate (liquid/solid) or 1 mg glucagon	1 mg glucagon i.m or i.v or 25 g dextrose i.v.	25 g dextrose i.v. or 1 mg glucagon i.v.	Mannitol (200 ml of 20 % solution) Dexamethasone (16–24 mg/day) High-flow oxygen Anticonvulsants Sedation Dextrose/insulin infusion Potassium infusion

Always give oral carbohydrate (20–40 g) when consciousness has been regained

FIGURE 5.1 Treatment of hypoglycemia; the complexity of treatment is governed primarily by duration of hypoglycemia

Severe hypoglycemia may require treatment with i.m. glucagon or i.v. dextrose (Fig. 5.1).

Alcohol consumption can interfere with symptomatic awareness of hypoglycemia and can also impair counterregulatory hormonal responses, while the features of hypoglycemia may be mistaken for inebriation. The frequency of mild hypoglycemia is increased following alcohol consumption, and delayed hypoglycemia occurring several hours after drinking is well recognized.

Morbidity of Hypoglycemia

Severe hypoglycemia can cause coma and seizures and can result in personal injury, including fractures, dislocations, and soft tissue injuries. It is less well appreciated that hypoglycemia can precipitate cardiovascular events through inducing myocardial ischemia and cardiac arrhythmias, and cerebrovascular lesions such as stroke and hemiplegia can occur. Fortunately, permanent brain damage is rare. The dangers of very strict glycemic control, with its increased risk of severe hypoglycemia, in a diabetic population which has a high risk of cardiovascular disease have been highlighted by the outcome of large trials, such as ACCORD and VADT, that examined the effect of strict glycemic control on cardiovascular outcomes in type 2 diabetes. Hypoglycemia while driving can cause road traffic accidents.

Fear of Hypoglycemia

Hypoglycemia is unpleasant and may be embarrassing or even humiliating but also can cause serious morbidity and may be life-threatening. Fear of hypoglycemia is therefore very common and not only affects people with diabetes but also their relatives. As a consequence, fear of hypoglycemia can modify behavior so that elevated blood glucose levels are preferred. Hypoglycemia has implications for driving, certain types of employment, and personal relationships and in some patients can lead to significant psychological problems.

Weight Gain

Undesirable weight gain is also an adverse effect of intensive therapy with insulin. Weight gain associated with insulin treatment, particularly when glycemic control is improved, is a major clinical problem. The underlying causes are decreased caloric loss through a reduction in glycosuria with better glycemic control, the anabolic effects of insulin on adipose tissue, a decreased metabolic rate, a decrease in leptin uptake, treatment of recurrent hypoglycemia with additional carbohydrate, and defensive eating to avoid the risk of hypoglycemia.

The association between increasing weight gain and insulin therapy has been shown in a number of large, prospective studies. In the Diabetes Control and Complications Trial (DCCT), the average weight gain of patients with type 1 diabetes in the intensive treatment arm was 5 kg. In the course of the United Kingdom Prospective Diabetes Study (UKPDS), those patients with type 2 diabetes who were treated with insulin had more than double the weight gain of those treated with glibenclamide (4.0 vs. 1.7 kg) despite equivalent levels of glycemic control; across all therapies, patients in the intensive-treatment group generally gained about 3.1 kg in weight compared with the those in the conventional-treatment group. In addition to weight gain being undesirable and contributing to insulin resistance, there is the added problem of the fear of gaining weight, which is a common problem in adolescent girls and young women, many of whom deliberately omit insulin doses to control their body weight.

Management of Weight Gain

Weight gain with insulin therapy is not inevitable, and being alert to the problem may partly help to avoid it. An adequate insulin regimen and lifestyle changes can help to minimize this side-effect of insulin therapy. Lifestyle interventions are an effective starting point, but patients need adequate professional support in planning and sticking to appropriate diet and exercise regimens—studies have shown that such interventions can be effective. Combination therapy of insulin with oral metformin is a further approach which may limit weight gain in some patients. There is some evidence that weight gain is less with the use of some long-acting insulin analogues—particularly insulin detemir.

Lipohypertrophy and Lipoatrophy

In the days of relatively impure animal insulins, the subcutaneous fat tissue at the site of insulin injection could disappear over time, leaving an unsightly indentation in the skin—so-called lipoatrophy. This was thought to be an allergic reaction to impurities in the insulin; it rarely occurs with modern insulins. By contrast, lipohypertrophy is a trophic reaction of subcutaneous adipose tissue to repeated injections of insulin into the same site. It can lead to erratic and delayed absorption of insulin and so to unpredictable glycemic excursions. Patients often find these areas unsightly, but they generally will gradually resolve if insulin is not injected into the affected area. Patients should be reminded of the need to rotate their injection sites.

Skin Infections

Although insulin injections could theoretically cause infection in subcutaneous tissues, it very rarely happens in practice, because insulin preparations contain an antiseptic. However, with continuous subcutaneous insulin infusion therapy (Chap. 3), the microfine subcutaneous catheter remains in place for several days. Local skin infection with erythema can result, but this risk is minimized if good hygiene is employed at the time of changing infusion sets and if the sets are changed after a maximum of 3 days.

Insulin Allergy

Very rarely, patients can develop a local urticarial reaction in response to an insulin injection. The hypersensitivity reaction is in itself not serious, but it is itchy and uncomfortable. The presumption is that this is an allergic response to an excipient in the insulin solution, rather than to the insulin itself. Antihistamines and topical steroids may be of benefit, but this is best managed by switching to another insulin.

Chapter 6
Intravenous Insulin

Administration of subcutaneous (s.c.) insulin poses potential problems for a patient who is acutely ill and unable to take oral glucose. The insulin will exert a hypoglycemic effect for several hours, but the rate of absorption is unpredictable in people who are shocked and have peripheral vasoconstriction. Intravenous (i.v.) insulin, by contrast, has a short half-life (2.5 min) and has to be given as a continuous infusion. This works immediately and its effects can be stopped by discontinuing the infusion; dose adjustments have an immediate effect. Insulin delivery by the i.v. route has several indications (Table 6.1), but it is often overprescribed—non-fasting patients are frequently and unnecessarily given i.v. insulin to control hyperglycemia in the absence of ketosis or hyperosmolality. In these situations, s.c. insulin or oral anti-diabetic medications should be used.

Because i.v. insulin lowers blood glucose rapidly, it is usual to coadminister a glucose-based intravenous crystalloid. Not only does the glucose prevent hypoglycemia, it also provides substrate to prevent catabolism. The insulin and glucose can be administered in the same infusion bag, along with potassium chloride (called a "GKI" regimen) or can be administered (with potassium) using separate infusion systems (an insulin "sliding scale" regimen or variable rate insulin infusion [VRII]). The *VRII* regimen is less labor-intensive and is suitable for patients with pronounced hyperglycemia. However, if the glucose infusion is interrupted, the continued infusion of unopposed insulin can provoke severe hypoglycemia, so careful

M.W.J. Strachan, B.M. Frier, *Insulin Therapy,*
DOI 10.1007/978-1-4471-4760-2_6,
© Springer-Verlag London 2013

TABLE 6.I Common indications for intravenous insulin

Perioperative control of blood glucose

Peripartum control of diabetes

Diabetic ketoacidosis

Hyperosmolar nonketotic coma

Strict glycemic control of prognostic benefit, e.g., critical care patients

Emergency management of hyperkalemia

monitoring of blood glucose concentrations and the infusions is essential. The *GKI regimen* is more labor-intensive and less suitable for markedly hyperglycemic patients. In addition, if used for more than 24 h, the high volume of i.v. glucose delivers a large hypotonic fluid load. However, if the infusion device fails, then both insulin and dextrose will cease simultaneously, limiting the risk of hypoglycemia.

The choice of insulin and glucose regimen is usually determined by the experience of the ward nursing staff, the anesthetist, and the local hospital protocols, but most centers now favor VRII.

> Intravenous insulin has a half-life of only 2.5 min; if an infusion is discontinued, hyperglycemia (and potentially ketosis) can quickly ensue.

Variable Rate Insulin Infusion Regimen

An insulin infusion is prepared by adding 50 units of soluble (regular) insulin to 0.9 % saline in a syringe to a total volume of 50 ml, so that 1 ml of the solution contains 1 unit of insulin. The dose is adjusted according to a sliding scale; an example is shown in Table 6.2.

Monitoring and Adjusting the VRII

Capillary blood glucose should be measured hourly. The doses prescribed in a VRII initially represent a "best guess" as to the

TABLE 6.2 Example of a VRII

BG (mmol/l)	Insulin infusion (soluble insulin units/h = ml/h)
>20.0	Discuss with diabetes team
17.1–20.0	6
14.1–17.0	5
11.1–14.0	4
9.0–11.0	3
7.1–9.0	2
4.1–7.0	1
<4[a]	0.5[a]

[a]Remember that people with type 1 diabetes will quickly become ketotic if i.v. insulin is discontinued for any appreciable length of time, so do not stop i.v. insulin for a prolonged period without close supervision. A zero rate is acceptable if the patient has remained on s.c. long-acting insulin

appropriate amount of insulin to infuse for a given blood glucose. Obese patients may require higher rates of insulin infusion, while thin patients may be more insulin-sensitive. It is vital that medical staff monitor the blood glucose response every 2–4 h because the VRII may require adjustment to ensure that blood glucose remains between 6 and 10 mmol/l (between 4 and 12 mmol/l is acceptable, however). If the insulin infusion rate has to be changed frequently and blood glucose is fluctuating widely, the sliding scale needs to be reviewed (Table 6.3). The frequency of monitoring can be reduced if blood glucose is stable and within the target range. Regrettably, in clinical practice the complexity of managing a VRII is often delegated to unskilled staff, with potentially adverse consequences, and is frequently misused in inexperienced hands.

If the capillary blood glucose is >12 mmol/l, blood or urine should also be checked for ketones.

Blood glucose responses should be reviewed every 2–4 h while using a VRII to determine whether insulin doses require adjustment.

TABLE 6.3 Hourly capillary glucose and insulin infusion rates in an individual patient

Clock time (h)	BG (mmol/l)	Insulin infusion (units soluble insulin/h = ml/h)
08.00	13.4	4
09.00	7.4	2
10.00	13.9	4
11.00	9.1	2

The insulin infusion rates are being adjusted every hour in response to fluctuating capillary blood glucose levels. The sliding scale should be revised to the following and reviewed after 2–4 h

BG (mmol/l)	Insulin infusion (units soluble insulin/h = ml/h)
>20.0	Discuss with diabetes team
17.1–20.0	6
14.1–17.0	5
7.1–14.0	3
4.1–7.0	1
<4[a]	0.5

Co-prescribing Glucose and Potassium with a VRII

Whenever i.v. insulin is infused, i.v. glucose is also necessary (unless significant hyperglycemia is present). This was traditionally provided as 5 or 10 % glucose, but increasingly 5 % glucose/0.45 % saline is preferred as a means of providing additional sodium. If a patient is volume-overloaded, 20 % glucose can be used, but is hypertonic and irritant to veins and local tissues, and should be administered via a central line.

The daily requirement for potassium is approximately 60 mmol/day. Glucose and insulin cause hypokalemia, and unless the patient is hyperkalemic (plasma potassium >5.5 mmol/l), i.v. potassium should also be administered continuously. The precise amount depends on the patient's plasma potassium (and total body potassium store). Glucose (both 5 and 10 % and 5/0.45 % saline) is available with pre-added potassium chloride (usually 10 mmol/500 ml bag [0.15 %] or 20 mmol/500 ml bag [or 0.3 %]), and these are safer to use than adding potassium separately.

The rate of the substrate infusion should be determined by the state of hydration of the patient, but most commonly 100–125 ml/h is prescribed. Plasma urea, electrolytes, and laboratory blood glucose should be measured daily.

> The KCl content of the intravenous fluids should be prescribed according to plasma K^+ concentration. Particular care is necessary in patients with renal impairment.

The insulin and substrate should be given through the same i.v. cannula, to avoid the danger of a blockage resulting in only one of the two drugs being administered. The insulin syringe should be attached to a giving set that incorporates a Y-connector with a one-way and antisiphon valves, to which the substrate infusion should be attached. The one-way valve prevents insulin being infused in a retrograde fashion into the substrate delivery set.

"Piggy-Backed" Fluids

Extra fluids are often required when a patient is receiving i.v. insulin and substrate. The patient may have intravascular volume depletion associated with intercurrent illness or from perioperative fluid loss. Giving alternate bags of glucose and saline or glucose and colloid should be avoided when a patient is receiving i.v. insulin. If additional fluids are required, these can be added ("piggy-backed") through a separate i.v. infusion line. This should be clearly specified to nursing staff—the simplest method is to have two separate and clearly labelled i.v. infusion charts, one for the each arm.

Anesthetists often prefer Hartmann's solution to 0.9 % sodium chloride because the latter may be associated with hyperchloremic acidosis. If a patient is to be maintained on i.v. insulin and glucose for more than 24 h, Hartmann's solution can be used to avoid hyponatremia. Acutely ill patients may require larger volumes of fluid and/or colloids.

> The glucose infusion is not intended to replace fluid volume; it is to maintain glycemic control.

> Do not alternate between administration of glucose and saline if a patient requires i.v. insulin and/or has diabetes.

Glucose, Potassium, Insulin (GKI) Regimen

A GKI regimen is managed using the principles described above, particularly with respect to additional i.v. fluids and monitoring. The standard initial prescription for a GKI regimen is:

- 500 ml 10 % glucose
- 10 mmol/l KCL (0.15 %)
- Insulin (usually 10 units of soluble insulin)
- Infusion at a rate of 100 ml/h

Determining the Starting Dose of Insulin in a GKI Regimen

As with a VRII, determining the initial starting dose of insulin in a GKI regimen can be difficult. The above regimen will provide approximately 50 units of insulin (five bags each containing 10 units) over a 24-h period. If a patient is taking very low or high doses of s.c. insulin, the dose will need adjustment.

If an obese patient requires more than 100 units per day, a standard GKI regimen is unlikely to suffice. When calculating the initial start-up dose of insulin, it is not simply a matter of dividing the total daily dose of insulin by 5, because the "standard" insulin dose that the patient usually administers was determined during normal health. If given during severe illness, this may cause suboptimal glycemic control. However, a calculation of the 5-hourly insulin infusion rate based on the patient's total daily requirement will give an approximate estimate of the likely insulin dose. It is better to err on the side of caution as hyperglycemia is less harmful to the sick patient in the short-term than severe hypoglycemia. Conversely, a thin patient whose daily insulin dose is low will need a much lower starting dose of insulin.

Adjusting a GKI Regimen

Capillary blood glucose should be monitored hourly, until stability is ensured. If blood glucose rises to >12 mmol/l, a new GKI regimen should be commenced with 4 units *MORE* insulin in the bag and capillary blood glucose rechecked within 1 h. If blood glucose falls to below 6 mmol/l, a new GKI bag should be commenced with 4 units *LESS* insulin and capillary blood glucose rechecked within 1 h. If blood glucose is <4 mmol/l at any stage, or the patient develops symptomatic hypoglycemia, GKI should be discontinued and 10 % dextrose commenced at 100 ml/h until blood glucose is >5 mmol/l; the GKI may then be restarted with appropriate adjustment of the insulin dose.

Chapter 7
Use of Insulin in Hospitals

In this chapter, the practical applications of managing insulin therapy in hospital inpatients are discussed, with emphasis on the peri-operative management of diabetes, the acutely ill patient with diabetes, and the diabetic emergencies associated with hyperglycemia.

Effects of Intercurrent Illness and Surgery on Diabetes

At any time approximately 20 % of people in an acute hospital have diabetes—more than double the number expected based on prevalence of diabetes in the adult population. People with diabetes suffer from intercurrent illness and require surgery in the same way as those without diabetes, but hospital admission may be more frequent because of diabetes-related problems (Table 7.1).

Intercurrent illness and surgery release inflammatory mediators and counterregulatory hormones (e.g., epinephrine, cortisol) that promote catabolism (Fig. 7.1). Insulin resistance increases, favoring breakdown of glycogen, lipids, and protein; in a patient with diabetes, this can provoke hyperglycemia and ketosis. To avoid this occurring, increased doses of insulin are required in those with insulin-treated diabetes, and insulin may have to be used temporarily in those taking antidiabetic medication. Hospitalized patients may be fasting

M.W.J. Strachan, B.M. Frier, *Insulin Therapy*,
DOI 10.1007/978-1-4471-4760-2_7,
© Springer-Verlag London 2013

TABLE 7.1 Diabetes-related reasons for admission to hospital

Medical

Ketoacidosis/hyperosmolar hyperglycemic states	Acute coronary syndrome
Hypoglycemia	Cerebrovascular accident
Renal failure	Limb infection/ischemia
Acute visual loss	Severe neuropathic pain

Surgical

Vitrectomy, cataract surgery	Coronary revascularization
Limb debridement/amputation	Carotid endarterectomy
Renal transplantation/vascular access	Limb revascularization
Pancreas/islet transplantation	Bariatric surgery[a]

[a]The management of diabetes in the time before and after bariatric surgery is highly specialized and is outwith the scope of this book; local protocols should be followed

or have poor oral intake; drugs which enhance catabolism, such as glucocorticoids, may be prescribed, and hospital-acquired infection presents well-documented risks.

Insulin requirements are significantly higher during intercurrent illness and following major surgery.

Target Glucose Concentrations

Despite the absence of randomized controlled trials, it is intuitive that good control of diabetes during serious illness should produce better outcomes, a premise supported by observational studies indicating that poor glycemic control in surgical patients is associated with greater mortality, risk of wound infections, and longer hospital stay. There is no consensus on the optimum glucose target for

Addressograph or Name, DOB, Unique identifier

BLOOD GLUCOSE MONITORING AND SUBCUTANEOUS INSULIN PRESCRIPTION CHART

Never omit insulin without consulting with medical staff

Usual insulin regimen:

If on intravenous insulin, please document hourly blood glucose readings on the intravenous insulin chart

DATE	BLOOD GLUCOSE (mmol/l)				INSULIN (units)												Hypoglycaemia: Time and Treatment
	Before Breakfast	Before Lunch	Before Tea	Before Bed	Before Breakfast			Before Lunch			Before Tea			Before Bed			
					Type/units	Prescribed by	Given by	Type/units	Prescribed by	Given by	Type/units	Prescribed by	Given by	Type/units	Prescribed by	Given by	
					UNITS			UNITS			UNITS			UNITS			
					UNITS			UNITS			UNITS			UNITS			
					UNITS			UNITS			UNITS			UNITS			
					UNITS			UNITS			UNITS			UNITS			
					UNITS			UNITS			UNITS			UNITS			
					UNITS			UNITS			UNITS			UNITS			
					UNITS			UNITS			UNITS			UNITS			

FIGURE 7.1 Subcutaneous insulin prescribing chart. Note the preprinted "units"

inpatients, but in essence hypoglycemia and extremes of hyperglycemia should be avoided. The American Diabetes Association has suggested a target range of blood glucose of 7.8–10 mmol/l for most patients and has stated that a lower target of 6.1–7.8 mmol/l may be appropriate in some patients (most notably those in a surgical critical care setting). Pragmatically a target blood glucose concentration of 6–10 mmol/l seems appropriate for most inpatients with diabetes; a range of 4–12 mmol/l is, however, generally considered acceptable control.

Prescribing and Adjusting Subcutaneous Insulin in Hospital

Errors in relation to the prescription of insulin are common on hospital wards. One-third of all inpatient medical errors that cause death within 48 h involve insulin. Subcutaneous (s.c.) insulin should only ever be prescribed on a specific "s.c. insulin prescription chart" (Fig. 7.1), and the prescription should be renewed every day depending on the previous day's glucose readings and the clinical condition of the patient. It is not an acceptable practice to prescribe fixed doses of insulin on a standard ward "drug kardex"; to do so risks the insulin being administered regardless of the prevailing blood glucose and removes the daily requirement for a medical practitioner to review the patient's glycemic control. Errors in relation to insulin can occur because of lack of knowledge on the part of the prescriber, or in the preparation or delivery of the insulin. Common errors are the wrong insulin being prescribed or administered (e.g., *Humalog* instead of *Humalog Mix 25*) or the insulin injection being inadvertently omitted or administered when the patient is not able to eat. Misreading the dose of prescribed insulin also occurs frequently, and the classic error in relation to this is when the letter "U" is misread as the number zero (0)—so while the doctor had prescribed "10u," the patient is given 100 units of insulin. To avoid this possibility, the dose of insulin should be written as a numerical figure; the term "units" or "U" should not be written (ideally it should be preprinted on the chart).

Adjustment of insulin and antidiabetic therapy on wards should be proactive, aiming for blood glucose values between 6 and 10 mmol/l. The principles of s.c. insulin dose adjustment in hospital are essentially the same as those discussed in Chap. 4. Persistent hyperglycemia and/or hypoglycemia should not be ignored, but it should be remembered that one-off lows or highs may have an explanation and do not require dose adjustment. Some examples of insulin dose adjustment are shown in Fig. 7.2.

Differences Between Type 1 and Type 2 Diabetes

People with type 1 diabetes have an absolute deficiency of insulin, and people with type 2 diabetes treated with diet and/ or tablets have a relative insulin deficiency, combined with insulin resistance. The former are at risk of developing ketoacidosis if they become catabolic or do not receive insulin, while this is seldom a problem with the latter. People with insulin-treated type 2 diabetes resemble type 1 diabetes, and their management should be similar. Individuals treated with glucagon-like peptide-1 (GLP-1) agonists (Exenatide and Liraglutide) may have an intermediate risk of ketosis. In this chapter patients have been subdivided into "insulin-treated" and "non-insulin-treated" groups.

Because of the very short half-life of i.v. insulin, there is a real risk that discontinuation of therapy (either deliberately or inadvertently) might result in ketosis. Accordingly, there is an increasing vogue to continue long-acting s.c. insulin therapy while patients are receiving i.v. insulin for whatever indication. This ensures that individuals have a reserve of insulin in their system and in theory should reduce the risk of ketosis if the i.v. insulin is stopped. Clearly, this is a situation that must be monitored closely to avoid hypoglycemia.

Patient A

	Blood glucose (mmol/l)							
Date	Before breakfast	Before lunch	Before tea	Before bed	Before breakfast Type/units	Before lunch Type/units	Before tea Type/units	Before bed Type/units
9/10	12.4	13.2	11.8	14.8	Novorapid 18 *units*	Novorapid 16 units	Novorapid 20 units	Glargine 24 units
10/10	13.8				*Novorapid 20 units*	*Novorapid 18 units*	*Novorapid 22 units*	*Glargine 26 units*

Comment: This patient has sustained hyperglycemia. If the patient has type 1 diabetes, ensure there is no ketonemia. Increased insulin dose is required—recommended doses are shown in italics. Given that all blood glucose levels are high, an alternative strategy would be to increase the dose of glargine by 6 units.

Patient B

	Blood glucose (mmol/l)							
Date	Before breakfast	Before lunch	Before tea	Before bed	Before breakfast Type/units	Before lunch Type/units	Before tea Type/units	Before bed Type/units
9/10	7.6	3.1	14.8	8.6	Novorapid 18 units	Novorapid 16 units	Novorapid 20 units	Glargine 24 units
10/10	6.2				*Novorapid 18 units*	*Novorapid 16 units*	*Novorapid 20 units*	*Glargine 24 units*

Comment: Check with nursing staff if there was any reason why the patient had an episode of hypoglycemia. If there was an obvious, non-recurring cause, for exmple, the patient had missed breakfast or had been sick, no adjustment to today's breakfast insulin is required. The pre-tea hyperglycaemia is probably a consequence of over-treatment of hypoglycemia, so rather than increasing the pre-lunch insulin by two units, it would probably be best to leave the insulin doses unchanged

Patient C

	Blood glucose (mmol/l)							
Date	Before breakfast	Before lunch	Before tea	Before bed	Before breakfast Type/units	Before lunch Type/units	Before tea Type/units	Before bed Type/units
9/10	7.6	12.4	14.8	8.6	Humalog Mix 25 18 *units*		Humalog Mix 25 20 *units*	
10/10	6.2				Humalog Mix 25 22 *units*		Humalog Mix 25 20 *units*	

Comment: The pre-lunch and pre-tea glucose levels are high. Increase the morning dose of the fixed mixture by 2–4 units

Patient D

	Blood glucose (mmol/l)							
Date	Before breakfast	Before lunch	Before tea	Before bed	Before breakfast Type/units	Before lunch Type/units	Before tea Type/units	Before bed Type/units
9/10	7.6	12.4	3.4	8.6	Humalog Mix 25 18 *units*		Humalog Mix 25 20 *units*	
10/10	6.2				Humalog Mix 50 18 units		Humalog Mix 25 20 units	

Comment: This is a tricky one! If this pattern of high pre-lunch and low pre-tea glucose is sustained, then increasing the dose of the 25/75 rapid-acting/isophane will correct the hyperglycemia but worsen the hypoglycemia. In this situation a switch to a 50/50 mixture may be preferable, that is, increasing the ratio of rapid-acting to isophane insulin

FIGURE 7.2 Examples of subcutaneous insulin dose adjustment

Patients treated with insulin and/or sulfonylureas can develop hypoglycemia; insulin-deficient patients are at risk of developing ketoacidosis.

Elective Peri-operative Management of Diabetes

The management of people with diabetes during the peri-operative period should follow simple principles.

Insulin-Treated Diabetes

It used to be a common practice to admit people with diabetes to hospital 2 or 3 days before elective surgery, "to optimize diabetes control." However, inpatient management of diabetes was often inferior to that obtained by the patient at home, and with increasing pressure on inpatient bed usage, most are now admitted either 1 day before surgery or on the morning of the procedure.

It is not always necessary to recourse to i.v. insulin during the peri-operative period, even for people with insulin-treated diabetes. If glycemic control is good and the surgery is relatively brief with a short period of postoperative fasting, delaying the morning rapid-acting s.c. insulin until after the procedure may be all that is necessary. By contrast, patients undergoing major surgery with an associated prolonged period of fasting usually require an i.v. insulin infusion.

It is a commonly held belief that "poorly controlled" diabetes is a reason to postpone elective surgery. Although there is no clear evidence that this will affect outcomes, glycemic control should be optimal if possible before planned surgery. Because many patients attend a preadmission clinic, this provides an opportunity to identify and address poor glycemic control.

Pre-operative Management

- Measure blood glucose (laboratory) and HbA1c at the preadmission clinic. If the HbA1c is >8.5 % (70 mmol/mol), the diabetes team should be asked if glycemic control can be improved before surgery. Other preadmission investigations (e.g., ECG and X-rays) should be performed as per local protocols.

- Liaise with the anesthetist and the surgical team so that the patient is either first or early on the list for surgery. Usually, the anesthetist will give instructions how the patient's diabetes is to be controlled peri-operatively. Advice can also be sought from the diabetes team.

- Encourage normal oral intake and prescribe usual medications on the day before surgery (unless the patient requires bowel preparation). Anesthetists vary in their guidance about fasting, but fasting times may include 6 h for food and 2 h for clear fluids (i.e. no milk and no carbonated drinks). Non-carbonated glucose drinks can be consumed up to 2 h before surgery, but it is essential that the anesthetist knows if these have been ingested.

- Monitor capillary blood glucose at least four times daily — if there are concerns about hypoglycemia or hyperglycemia, more frequent monitoring should be performed.

- Administer s.c. insulin as usual on the day before surgery. The only caveat to this is that the evening or bedtime insulin dose should be reduced by 20 % if the patient is prone to developing morning hypoglycemia.

- When the patient is taking oral antidiabetic agents, in combination with insulin, their administration should be managed according to the principles in the section on "non-insulin-treated diabetes."

It is not usually necessary to start i.v. insulin on the night before elective surgery.

Minor Surgery

When immediate postoperative resumption of oral intake is likely and the patient is placed early on the morning operation list, the following protocol may be used:

- Omit breakfast and the morning and lunchtime doses of rapid-acting insulin.
- Morning doses of long-acting insulins (*glargine*, *detemir*, *degludec*, *Insulatard*, or *Humulin I*) may be administered in their usual dose (providing the patient is not prone to "graze" during the day).
- If the patient is on a twice daily fixed mixture, halve the morning dose of insulin.
- The morning doses of other antidiabetic medications should be omitted, though Metformin and Pioglitazone can be given as usual (except in the cases of Metformin if the patient is going to receive radiological contrast).
- Check capillary blood glucose hourly from 8 a.m.
- Take no further action if the blood glucose remains between 4 and 12 mmol/l. VRII may be required if blood glucose rises above this range. I.v. glucose will be required if the patient is hypoglycemic.
- Postoperatively, s.c. insulin is given with food. The diabetes team can advise about the type of insulin and dose—but usually it will be a short-acting insulin or a fixed mixture and the dose will depend on the prevailing capillary glucose, the size of the meal, and the patient's sensitivity to insulin (which may be inferred from the patient's usual mealtime doses of insulin and body weight; see below).

Major Surgery

If the patient is undergoing major surgery and/or immediate resumption of oral intake after surgery is not planned, the following protocol should be used:

- The patient should be first on the operation list (preferably morning).

- Omit breakfast and the morning dose of insulin and other antidiabetic therapies. A morning dose of a long-acting insulin analogue (*glargine*, *detemir* and *degludec*) may be given.
- VRII should be commenced on the morning of surgery. The precise timing will usually be determined by the anesthetist but is usually at 8 a.m. or on arrival in theatre. If the patient is very hyperglycemic, the glucose infusion could be deferred until the VRII has lowered the blood glucose to <14 mmol/l, but this has to be monitored carefully to ensure the patient does not become hypoglycemic.
- Aim to maintain blood glucose between 6 and 10 mmol/l in the peri-operative period.

Re-establishing Subcutaneous Insulin

Re-establishing Subcutaneous insulin postoperatively can be difficult; it is clearly undesirable to give the patient s.c. insulin only for them to vomit after eating and then be at risk of hypoglycemia for several hours. Eating should be commenced while VRII and substrate are still in place. If a small dose of s.c. short-acting insulin is given with the first food, this should prevent a high preprandial glucose.

> VRII should not be discontinued until oral ingestion of food has been safely re-established.

When short-acting insulin is administered s.c., it takes time to exert its glucose-lowering effect. If i.v. insulin (which has a very short half-life) is discontinued too soon after commencing s.c. insulin, this may risk promoting hyperglycemia and even ketosis. Therefore, it should normally be stopped 1 h after the s.c. insulin injection. The VRII should not be stopped until the patient is eating and drinking normally.

The type of insulin to administer will depend on the patient's usual regimen and the time of day. If the patient is on a basal-bolus regimen, they should receive their usual "bolus"

TABLE 7.2 Converting intravenous to subcutaneous insulin

Estimation of dose from intravenous insulin requirements

Calculate the average hourly rate over the preceding 6 h

Multiply by 20[a] to get an average daily total

If using a basal-bolus regimen, give 50 % of the daily total as basal and divide the remaining 50 % between three bolus doses

If using a fixed mixture, give 60 % of the daily total in the morning and 40 % in the evening

Estimation of dose from weight

Type 2 diabetes 0.5–0.7 units/kg/day

Type 1 diabetes 0.3–0.5 units/kg/day

Split the daily total according to the insulin regimen, as above

[a]Multiply by 20 rather than 24 to reduce the risk of hypoglycemia

insulin before the appropriate meal. If the patient is on twice daily injections of a fixed mixture of insulin, this should be administered if the food to be eaten is breakfast or the evening meal. At lunchtime, the patient may be given a rapid-acting insulin analogue or a short-acting soluble insulin and their usual insulin given with their evening meal. If this additional dose of short-acting insulin is being given at lunchtime, it is important to indicate that this is an isolated injection on a single occasion, so that this is not repeated inappropriately on subsequent days. If there is doubt about what the patient will be able to eat, the s.c. insulin can be injected *after* their meal.

The s.c. insulin doses administered will depend on the prevailing capillary blood glucose, the amount of food to be eaten, and the patient's sensitivity to insulin. Most commonly, patients tend to be prescribed the same dose of insulin that they were receiving before admission to hospital, but clearly intercurrent illness may have significantly altered their insulin sensitivity (e.g., sensitivity will be enhanced by significant weight loss and reduced by a systemic inflammatory response). Estimation of the s.c. dose can be estimated from the preceding i.v. insulin requirements or from the patient's weight (Table 7.2).

Non-insulin-Treated Diabetes

Patients with well-controlled type 2 diabetes, managed with diet and/or oral antidiabetic agents, require careful monitoring of blood glucose alone during the peri-operative period. I.v. insulin is required only if postoperative fasting is prolonged or if glycemic control is very poor, for example, blood glucose values consistently >12 mmol/l.

Pre-operative Management

- Measure laboratory blood glucose and HbA1c at the pre-admission clinic. If the HbA1c is >8.5 % (70 mmol/mol), the diabetes team can be asked if they will optimize glycemic control before elective surgery. Sometimes s.c. insulin therapy may be required. Other preadmission investigations (e.g., ECG and X-rays) should be performed as per the local protocol.
- Liaise with the anesthetist and surgical list manager so that the patient is first (or early) on the list. Fasting requirements should be as for insulin-treated diabetes.
- If the patient is on a long-acting sulfonylurea, for example, glibenclamide, this should be changed to a shorter-acting preparation, for example, glipizide or gliclazide, at least 5 days before surgery. If this has not been changed, the longer-acting sulfonylureas should be omitted the evening before surgery, to minimize the risk of hypoglycemia.
- Metformin can be administered on the morning of surgery, providing the patient is not going to require i.v. radiological contrast. Pioglitazone can also be administered on the morning or surgery, as usual.
- Other oral antidiabetic agents, such as meglitinides and gliptins, should be omitted on the morning of surgery, as should injectable GLP-1 therapies.
- Check capillary blood glucose at the bedside, 2 hourly before surgery. If blood glucose is >12 mmol/l, commence VRII insulin and manage in same way as the patient with

insulin-treated diabetes. A higher dose of insulin is usually required.

- Avoid glucose-containing infusions and check capillary blood glucose 2 hourly.

Postoperative Management

- Antidiabetic therapy should be recommenced when oral feeding is reestablished. Metformin has been associated with lactic acidosis in the postoperative period. Risk factors include hypoxia, volume depletion, cardiac failure, and renal impairment. Metformin should not be restarted if any of these precipitating factors are present, and serum creatinine should be <150 μmol/l or estimated glomerular filtration rate (eGFR) less than 35 ml/min/1.73 m^2.
- If blood glucose is elevated postoperatively despite optimal antidiabetic therapy, s.c. insulin may be required.

Bowel Preparation and Endoscopy/ Colonoscopy

Patients who are to undergo colonoscopy or colorectal surgery usually have to take bowel preparation and clear fluids on the day before the procedure/surgery and have a modified low-residue diet for the preceding 1–2 days. This may affect glycemic control adversely but is rarely an indication for admission to hospital and i.v. insulin therapy. Patients should be given written instructions about what food and fluids they can and cannot eat and how to manage their insulin and other antidiabetic therapies.

Acute Intercurrent Illness and Diabetes

At the time of commencing insulin, written instructions should be given about what to do during intercurrent illness (sick-day rules), and these should be reinforced regularly

TABLE 7.3 Sick-day rules for people with type 1 diabetes

Capillary blood glucose should be estimated at least every 2 h
If capillary blood glucose is >12 mmol/l, check urine or blood for ketones
Plenty of clear fluids should be drunk to avoid dehydration
If food cannot be consumed, glucose-containing fluids should be ingested as an alternative
Insulin administration should not be stopped
Usually, insulin doses need to be INCREASED by 25–50 %
If vomiting or hyperketonemia or ketonuria is persistent, contact doctor or diabetes team

(Table 7.3). Patients fear hypoglycemia and will often omit or reduce insulin doses during intercurrent illness, when their oral intake is diminished. Reducing or omitting insulin at a time when insulin requirements are increased risks the development of severe hyperglycemia and ketosis. Although people with type 2 diabetes are at less risk of ketosis, this does occasionally occur, and they may be taking nephrotoxic medications such as angiotensin receptor inhibitors, which increase the risk of acute renal failure during a dehydrating illness.

> Insulin doses need to be increased, NOT reduced, during intercurrent illness.

Sick-Day Rules for Inpatients

The "sick-day rules" for patients also represent sound advice for junior doctors treating inpatients with diabetes. Persistent hyperglycemia should be treated. If the patient has insulin-treated diabetes, it is important to ensure they are not ketotic. Blood ketones are more useful to assess ketone status than urinary ketones. Venous bicarbonate is a useful initial guide to assessing acid–base status and if normal avoids the need for blood gas sampling.

If the patient is able to eat or drink and is not ketoacidotic, dose adjustment of oral antidiabetic therapy or s.c. insulin may suffice. However, Metformin should be discontinued in patients with renal impairment, acute hypoxia, heart failure, and/or liver disease. Pioglitazone is contraindicated in heart failure, and gliptins and GLP-1 analogues are contraindicated in renal impairment. If oral antidiabetic medications have to be discontinued or hyperglycemia persists despite maximal doses of these agents, s.c. insulin may have to be started.

Additional doses of s.c. insulin are often given to treat isolated hyperglycemia. This is treating a glucose value, not the patient. If the patient is ketotic and/or dehydrated, immediate treatment of hyperglycemia is justified but should be with i.v. insulin and fluids. However, if the patient is "well" and is eating and drinking normally, adjustment of s.c. insulin and/or antidiabetic therapy may be sufficient.

> Isolated hyperglycemia seldom requires urgent treatment with extra insulin outside usual prescription times.

I.v. insulin is indicated if the patient is not able to eat and drink or hyperglycemia is associated with ketosis or significant metabolic derangement. Typical scenarios would include a patient admitted with an acute abdomen who may be significantly dehydrated but oral fluids will be withheld. An elderly patient with insulin-treated diabetes and pneumonia may be unable to take oral food or fluids, and i.v. insulin may be required to maintain glycemic control. When prescribing fluids, the same principles should apply as for peri-operative management.

Hypoglycemia

Intercurrent illness is not solely about hyperglycemia and ketosis. Hypoglycemia is a major risk for inpatients treated with insulin and/or sulfonylureas. Patients may dislike hospital food, may have a poor appetite or be anorectic, or may simply miss a meal when they are away from the ward for an investigation or procedure. Hypoglycemia is potentially dangerous and should be avoided.

A particular hazard is the patient with poorly controlled type 1 diabetes, who is ostensibly requiring large doses of insulin. While people with type 1 diabetes may occasionally miss an injection of insulin, some with a high HbA1c >10 % (86 mmol/mol) may be deliberately omitting several doses, which they conceal from their physician. If unrecognized, increasing doses of insulin are prescribed and administered in hospital and provoke severe hypoglycemia. Admission to hospital may ensure that a patient is given all of their usual prescribed oral medication, which is in excess of their requirements.

> Persistent hyperglycemia and/or episodes of hypoglycemia require action by adjusting insulin and antidiabetic therapy.

Remember the Patient!

People who have been taking insulin for many years may become irritated when hospital staff try to alter their usual insulin therapy. They often know more about diabetic management than nonspecialist healthcare professionals. However, this assumed knowledge may be misplaced, and the effects of intercurrent illness or the impact of nondiabetic therapies on blood glucose may not be understood. When modifying a patient's treatment for diabetes, it is often useful to discuss the proposed changes with the patient. Specialist input may be necessary, particularly if the patient objects to the proposed changes. The patient's own treatments for hypoglycemia should not be removed without good reason.

Diabetic Ketoacidosis (DKA) and Hyperosmolar Hyperglycemic State (HHS)

All hospitals should have established protocols for the management of DKA and HHS that are readily available to junior medical staff. In general, problems in the management of DKA and HHS are usually a consequence of the protocol not being followed! Discussion of the pathophysiology, precipitants, and management of DKA and HHS is beyond the scope of this book, but the key issues regarding the prescription of i.v. insulin are addressed.

> When treating a patient with DKA or HHS, follow the hospital protocol.

Should a VRII, GKI, or Fixed-Rate Infusion of Insulin Be Used?

In principle, any of these modalities could be used, but a GKI is probably best avoided as administering i.v. glucose is undesirable when a patient is very hyperglycemic. Therefore, all DKA and HHS protocols mandate the use of i.v. saline initially to rehydrate the patient. I.v. glucose should be commenced only when blood glucose is <14 mmol/l. As with the peri-operative protocols, it will invariably be necessary to "piggy back" saline onto the glucose infusion, that is, the patient is still likely to be volume depleted and will need more i.v. fluid. Glucose and saline should not be given alternately—the glucose and insulin infusion should be infused into one arm with the saline infusion into the other. Most people with DKA and HHS have a profound total body potassium deficit; the local protocol for potassium replacement should be followed with care.

Is the Prescription for the VRII the Same as for Peri-operative Patients?

The peri-operative VRII must NOT be used in the management of patients with DKA or HHS. In DKA, ketogenesis often continues even though blood glucose has fallen to <14 mmol/l. High doses of insulin are required to inhibit ketogenesis, and in practice, this means that the insulin infusion rate should not be lowered below 3units/h. The peri-operative VRII is inappropriate for use in DKA because when blood glucose declines to below 10 mmol/l, lower doses of insulin will be infused. Thus, in DKA, 6 units/h of insulin should be prescribed until blood glucose is <14 mmol/l. At that stage, the insulin infusion rate should be reduced to 3 units/h and i.v. glucose prescribed as above. The target blood glucose range is 9–14 mmol/l. If higher doses of insulin are required to maintain this level, the infusion rate should be adjusted. If blood glucose falls below this target, the rate or concentration of the glucose infusion should be increased. High doses of insulin are prescribed to inhibit ketogenesis, and high doses of glucose are administered to permit the use of high-dose insulin. The blood glucose should be measured frequently and simple, commonsense adjustments made to the insulin and glucose prescriptions as required. When the serum bicarbonate has returned to normal, ketones are no longer detectable and the patient is eating and drinking, s.c. rapid-acting insulin can be reintroduced, as for peri-operative patients. As with these patients, many specialists now recommend that long-acting s.c. analogue insulins should be continued during i.v. insulin therapy for DKA.

An alternative to the VRII regimen specified above is to administer a *fixed-rate infusion* of insulin at 0.1 unit/kg/h. Fixed rates have long been advocated in pediatric practice and increasingly are finding favor in adult medical practice. The theoretical advantage of the fixed-rate infusion is that it takes into account the inherent insulin sensitivity of the individual, which is not effected with the VRII regimen. This may be an issue in the very obese and in people with insulin resistance states, such as pregnancy.

Patients with HHS are extremely dehydrated, but are seldom significantly ketoacidotic. Plasma sodium and glucose need to be lowered gradually to avoid rapid shifts in fluid, which may precipitate neurological complications. I.v. fluids alone help to lower blood glucose, and many protocols advocate using 0.45 % saline. Insulin infusion rates are also lower in HHS, and many specialists advocate an initial infusion rate of 3 units/h. Patients with HHS should be managed in a high dependency unit with close supervision by experienced medical staff.

> High doses of insulin are required to inhibit ketogenesis; a zero-rate insulin infusion should never be prescribed in treating DKA.

Insulin Pumps

As described in Chap. 3, continuous subcutaneous insulin infusion (CSII) therapy is a highly effective method of managing type 1 diabetes. The use of this therapy is steadily increasing, and some patients will inevitably be admitted to hospital with diabetes or nondiabetes-related illness. In general, the principles of management of patients receiving CSII do not differ from others with type 1 diabetes, but the following key points are important:

- Patients on CSII have no depot of basal insulin so if the pump is disconnected or discontinued for any appreciable length of time, ketoacidosis can develop. If CSII is discontinued for more than 1 h, insulin must be administered by another route — either s.c. or i.v. — and it may take several hours for s.c. administered insulin to reach an effective therapeutic level.
- Many patients prefer to use their pump during a hospital admission, and most patients using CSII are well informed about insulin management. They will almost certainly know much more about using a pump than the hospital staff providing their care! It is often entirely reasonable for patients to continue using their pump, but close liaison with the hospital diabetes team is advised.
- If a patient is to undergo major surgery, then the patient should be managed with VRII in the conventional way and the pump discontinued when the infusion is commenced.

- For minor surgery, it may be possible to continue with the pump, but this needs prior discussion with the anesthetist and patient.
- The pump should be disconnected before X-ray, CT, and MRI investigations.

Never discontinue an insulin pump for more than one hour without ensuring that an alternative means of replacing insulin has been provided.

Index

M.W.J. Strachan, B.M. Frier, *Insulin Therapy,*
DOI 10.1007/978-1-4471-4760-2,
© Springer-Verlag London 2013